D1559863

THE ORIGINS OF GENERAL NURSING

The Origins of
General Nursing

CHRISTOPHER J. MAGGS

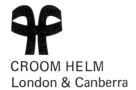

CROOM HELM
London & Canberra

© 1983 Christopher J. Maggs
Croom Helm Ltd, Provident House, Burrell Row,
Beckenham, Kent BR3 1AT

British Library Cataloguing in Publication Data

Maggs, Christopher J.
    The origins of general nursing.
    1. Nursing — History
    I. Title
    610.73'09   RT31

    ISBN 0-7099-1734-1

Printed and bound in Great Britain by
Biddles Ltd, Guildford and King's Lynn

CONTENTS

TABLES

This book is dedicated to June, Joseph and Hannah:
and with thanks to Margaret.

This is a study of the first generation of general hospital trained nurses in England, who emerged from their training hospitals between 1881 and 1914 to infiltrate and dominate the entire nursing world for the next half-century. "Illness creates dependency", as Brian Abel-Smith has pointed out,[1] and this first cadre of general nurses exploited that dependency to develop and maintain an occupational supremacy which has pervaded the profession since: after the hiccups of the First World War and its need for more nurses than the civilian system could provide,[2] general nursing came to reign supreme in the occupation and its representatives decided the structures of nursing until the present day.[3] That superiority was built upon the early decisions and pragmatic developments which situated nurse training in the hospital rather than, say, in the community: the growth and importance of the general hospitals in medicine and medical care depended on creating a large labour force of competent nurse practitioners to staff them, and the existence of this labour force, which needed training to become competent, in turn stimulated the developments within the general hospitals.

General hospital nurses were those nurses working in, or trained by, the voluntary and Poor Law general hospitals and infirmaries; however, what constituted a general nurse or indeed a general hospital is not immediately obvious. Some hospitals provided medical, surgical and childrens' treatments, some offered provision for gynaecological care, while others did not admit either children or women suffering from strictly female complaints to their wards. A few of the general hospitals had fever and other specialist wards, although most tended to treat any such cases on the general wards themselves. The only basic similarity between the range of general hospitals was that they all provided care divided between the two major branches of medicine then extant; i.e. beds were provided for use by physicians and surgeons and patients were cared for as medical or surgical cases. Since the statutes of many of the early voluntary hospitals specifically excluded certain

1

conditions from being treated within the wards of the hospitals, notably gynaecological and post-partum conditions, and the contemporary virulence of contagious and infectious conditions tended to inhibit their admission to such hospitals, what constituted a general hospital was largely an historical development which also reflected local needs.[4]

Since nurse training reflected medical training and the division between medicine and surgery, general nurses ought, therefore, to be nurses trained solely in the care of patients in general hospitals: however, as we shall see, general hospital nurses were taught a core curriculum which was to provide them with a range of skills across the nursing spectrum. The general trained nurse came, therefore, to resemble not so much the hospital consultant as the emerging general practitioner, who indeed saw the new nurse as a direct competitor. General hospital trained nurses, then, were nurses who had learnt a basic set of skills and knowledge which had been evolved by that section of the occupation to provide them with universal application. The general nurse, once trained, could therefore go anywhere in the world of nursing and health armed with this universal expertise and carry out any of the multifarious tasks and skills required of a nurse, specialist or generalist.

This book attempts to trace the emergence of that first generation of general nurses in order to show how they came to dominate nursing in England for so long, not necessarily as individuals, since this is not a study of personalities, but collectively as representatives of the new order. This study is not directly about the process of professionalisation,[5] nor about the "politics of nursing"[6] nor is it an attempt to find the roots of nursing in antiquity,[7] or describe "ministering angels" at work in the world.[8] This present work is concerned with the way in which women chose and were chosen to be general nurses and the consequences that their decisions subsequently had for nursing.

We shall, therefore, be concerned with an examination of recruitment to general nurse training and with that training itself, as it helped to instil in the recruit values which she carried over into her post-training experiences and which led her to see herself, and to others seeing her, as a member of a group at the apex of the occupation, if not as a member of an exclusive elite. That superiority will be examined through an analysis of post-general training work patterns and by reference to some popular images of contemporary nurses.

This present study, then, will address itself directly to a deliberate omission from what has since become, to the occupation if not to historians, "the history" of nursing[9]: it will attempt to repair the historiographical consequences of Professor Abel-Smith's statement that in his study

> no attempt is made to provide a history of nursing techniques or of nursing as an activity or skill.

> Little is said about what it was like at different
> times to nurse, or to receive nursing care. What
> the nurse was taught, who taught her, who examined
> her are all questions which are left unanswered.[10]

This book should be seen, therefore, as complementary to
that written over twenty years ago by Abel-Smith; together
they will help the historian understand how it was that the
general trained nurse came to occupy such a central position
in nursing. They are also complementary in that this study
concentrates on the experiences of the nurses themselves
rather than the leadership or reformers of the profession, and
thus it offers to redress some of the imbalance within the
historiography of nursing. While its sample population is
small, it is intended also to stimulate or encourage others to
look more closely at the micro-historical event as contribut-
ing to macro-historical explanations: local studies of nurse
training schools and hospitals need not be antiquarian but important case-studies for the history of nursing and healthcare
provisions, and for the history of women in general.

NOTES

1. B. Abel-Smith, A History of the Nursing Profession
(Heinemann, London, 1960) (1975 edition), p. 1. See also J.
Vaizey, Scenes from Institutional Life (Faber and Faber,
London, 1959), "For ... Kay and Richard Titmus who agree that
Institutions give inadequate people what they want - power",
Dedication, np.
2. The numbers of casualties and widespread theatres of
conflict required significant numbers of nurses which a
lengthy training programme would obstruct: hence, the short
training in basic nursing given to women in the Voluntary Aid
Detachments; For an overview, see Abel-Smith, Nursing Profession, pp. 83-88.
3. Abel-Smith, Nursing Profession, Chapters X, XI and
XVI.
4. J. Woodward, To Do The Sick No Harm: A Study of the
British Voluntary Hospital System to 1875 (Routledge and Kegan
Paul, London, 1974) (1978 edition), pp. 36-74.
5. For recent discussions of nursing and professionalisation, see C. Davies, 'Continuities in the Development of
Hospital Nursing in Britain', Journal of Advanced Nursing, 2,
1977, M. Carpenter, 'The New Managerialism and Professionalism
in Nursing' in M. Stacey et al (eds.), Health Care and the
Division of Labour (Croom Helm, London, 1977); C. Davies,
'Professionalizing Strategies as Time- and Culture-Bound. The
Case of American Nursing circa 1893', unpublished paper read
to B.S.A. Medical Sociology Conference, York, 1978.
6. Abel-Smith, Nursing Profession, p. xi.
7. A common theme in studies of nursing: see, for

example, M. Baly, <u>Nursing and Social Change</u> (Heinemann, London 1973); P. Kalisch and B. Kalisch, <u>The Advance of American Nursing</u> (Little, Boston, U.S.A. 1978); J. Iveson-Iveson, 'The Spiritual Side', <u>Nursing Mirror</u>, 17 March 1982, p. 22-24.

8. S. Bingham, <u>Ministering Angels</u> (Van Nos Reinhold, London, 1980).

9. C. Davies, 'Where Next for Nursing History?', <u>Nursing Times</u>, 22 May 1980, p. 922.

10. Abel-Smith, <u>Nursing Profession</u>, p. xi.

Chapter 1

THE BACKGROUND

All professions are conspiracies against the laity.[1]

Introduction: The revolution begins
The emergence of a new order of nursing, which set the general
trained nurse at the pinnacle of the heterogeneous occupation,
dates practically from the spread of hospital nurse training
after the 1880's throughout the expanding general hospital
network, voluntary and Poor Law alike.[2] Some reformers claimed
that it was the direct influence of Florence Nightingale which
had resulted in the establishment of a trained profession and
a trained elite within it: thus

> until 40 years ago there was practically no trained
> nursing in this country, and no trained nurses ....
> Since the Crimea War, a better class of women have
> entered the calling; they have gradually introduced
> many much needed improvements in the greater care of
> the sick and greater attention to them and the
> method of their dietary.[3]

Others, perhaps closer to the day-to-day problems of providing medical and nursing services within the hospitals, men
like Sir Henry Burdett, Bart., one-time Secretary of the Sea-
men's Hospital, Greenwich and before that Queen's Hospital,
Birmingham, saw the emergence of 'modern' nursing inextricably
linked to the expansion of the general hospital system itself.
[4] For such observers a shorter time-scale for the developments
within nursing was a more accurate description of events.
Asked by a member of the Select Committee on the Registration
of Nurses (1904) whether he agreed that "the nursing profession has become of vital importance in the last few years?",
Burdett agreed that it had been steadily improving but that he
dated that 'revolution' from the 1880's only.[5]
Whether the revolution dates from the 1860's and the influence of Nightingale via her 'nightingales' at St. Thomas's
Hospital, or from the institutional changes after 1880 which
Burdett had so frequently described and contributed to, all
contemporaries agreed that nursing had undergone fundamental

5

change by the closing years of the nineteenth-century, and
that that change had been for the better. This developmental
approach argued, as did the reformers rhetoric, for a transition from an unenlightened past to a more desirable future.[6]
While some reformers, notably those in favour of State regulation of nurses, felt that the revolution was not progressing
at a quick enough pace, all tended to see the instigation of a
formal training scheme as a crucial development in the campaign to raise nursing standards and the status of nurses.[7]
Before looking at that training we shall need to describe some
of the influences on the emergence of general nursing in the
period 1881 - 1914.

The growth of hospitals and the need for nurses

As long as there have been hospitals, there have been hospital
nurses working in them, lay and religious women who kept the
patients and their surroundings clean, gave out food and medicines and who were enjoined to "follow the Physician's orders
duly".[8] The lay members of this workforce were invariably
widowed (occasionally married) women who have been long
characterised, if not caricatured, as being little more than
domestic servants of a rather rough and coarse type.[9]

In 1800 there were about 4,000 general hospital beds, and
out of a total population of approximately ten millions (Great
Britain) only 30,000 persons ever became in-patients (1801).[10]
The consequent need for nurses was also low, even if the
nurse/patient ratio had been close to that found at the end of
the nineteenth-century when it was 1:6.[11] Hospital nurses as
an identifiable occupational grouping, distinct from religious
orders and from other hospital 'servants' only emerge with the
expansion of the general and specialist hospital sector from
the 1880's onwards.

Statistics relating to the growth of hospital provision
in the nineteenth-century are somewhat crude and are especially so when we are concerned with such indicators of healthcare provision as bed-occupancy. In 1861 there were 23 voluntary teaching hospitals and 130 voluntary general hospitals in
England and Wales, providing about 12,000 beds; by 1891 this
bed provision had increased to 22,000 and to 37,000 by 1921.
At the same time the provision of sick-beds in the Poor Law
service increased, both as beds on sickwards of existing
Unions and in the increasing number of separate infirmaries
administered by the Poor Law Local Government Board. In 1891
there were 12,000 beds in separate Poor Law infirmaries rising
to 41,000 in 1911. As Table 1.1 shows, there was a massive expansion, approximately 140%, in the total provision of general
hospital beds in the two sectors combined between 1861 and
1921, with the greatest increase occuring between 1891 and
1911.

This expansion was accompanied by a similar one in the
smaller or more specialised areas of hospital care, fever and

6

Table 1.1: The Number of Beds in Hospitals by Type of
Institution, England and Wales 1861 - 1921

Hospitals	1861	1891	1911	1921
Teaching Voluntary	5291	7226	8284	9584
General Voluntary	6658	15184	21651	27443
General Public [a]	-	12138	40927	37840
Totals General Voluntary and Public Hospitals	6658	27322	62578	65283

Source: R. Pinker, English Hospital Statistics 1861 -
1938 (Heinemann, London, 1966), p. 61 Table
IX (abridged).

a.   Includes an unknown number of chronic sick

smallpox hospitals, sanatoria, asylums and cottage hospitals,
etc., all of which soaked up a percentage of the available
nursing population, trained and untrained. In 1883, for example, Burdett had recommended about 150 cottage hospitals to
his predominantly middle-class readership; by 1896 the number
of recommended cottage hospitals had risen to over 300.[12] Some
of these hospitals were tiny with only two or three beds;
others had up to 100 beds. Even the smallest employed at least
one day-nurse and sometimes one night-nurse, and normally the
day-nurse at least was required to be 'trained'. Such hospitals, to which we might add some 'fringe' establishments associated with, for example, homeopathy or other contemporary
fashionable treatment regimes, made inroads into the available
nursing population and gave considerable impetus for it to increase.
    Given the difficulties inherent in Census data, at least
until 1921, and the lack of firm evidence from the hospitals
themselves, it is difficult to know precisely how many hospital nurses there were in the early period.[13] Taking a crude
nurse/patient ratio of 1:6 and the estimates made by others of
bed-provisions throughout the period, we can estimate that
less than 1,000 women worked as hospital nurses (religious and
lay) before 1861; by the end of the century our estimate would
suggest that there were approximately 12,500 nurses working in
general hospitals.
    Burdett's evidence on the Select Committee on the Regis-
tration of Nurses (1905) gave figures of 11,038 nurses employed in voluntary hospitals, to which need be added those
working in the Poor Law service, approximately 5,000.[14] The
total number of women returned as nurses in any category in

Table 1.2: Number of Nurses Employed, and Percentage
Increase in number employed, in England
and Wales 1861 - 1911

Year	Numbers	Inter-Censal % Increase
1861	24821	-
1871	28417	14.5
1881	35175[a]	23.8
1891	53057[b]	50.8
1901	64214	21.0
1911	77060	20.0
1861 - 1911	52239	210.5

Source: L. Holcombe, <u>Victorian Ladies at Work</u> (David
and Charles, Newton Abbot, 1973), Appendix
Section 2, Tables 2a and 2b, pp. 204-5.

a. "Described in this census report as 'subor-
dinate medical service'".
b. "This figure includes those returned as midwives. However, they were not a relatively
large number in 1881, 2,646 and in 1901,
3055".

Table 1.3: Total Number of Nurses (Male and Female)
in Full-time equivalents and the total
population, in England and Wales 1901-1931

	1901	1921	1931
Total Population (thousands)	32528	37887	39952
Nurses in Full-time Equivalents	(69200)[a]	122804[a]	153843
No of Nurses per thousand	(2.13)	3.25	3.85

Source: B. Abel-Smith, <u>A History of the Nursing Profes-
sion</u> (Heinemann, London, 1960) (1975 edition),
Table 1, p. 256.
a. Includes 5,700 male nurses in 1901 and 11,303
male nurses in 1921.

our period are presented in Tables 1.2 and 1.3: less than half of all nurses, therefore, worked in the hospitals of England and Wales at the turn of the century, and of those working in the general hospitals three-quarters were probationers (nurses in training) and only a quarter were qualified and trained nurses. Hospital nursing, and general hospital nursing especially, while remaining a small part of an expanding occupation, appears to have grown at least coincidentally with the growth of hospitals.

It was not just numbers which were required to meet the demands of the expanding hospital network; the workforce was being asked to actively contribute to medical care, to play its part in creating an efficient hospital regime and especially to help cut costs. Nursing of the new order would involve antiseptic and aseptic techniques; careful and consciencious administrations of treatments and drugs; working to an ordered day with shifts and hierarchies of functions, and absolute trustworthiness, both to the administrators and to the doctors.

For many contemporaries, engaged as they were in developing the new system of nursing, the new generation of nurses cared for their patients "better" and at a "quicker pace". "Medical treatment was implemented more reliably and efficiently" by the new nurses, which led directly to a reduction in mortality rates, even if that contribution consisted of carrying out the orders of the doctors rather than developing any form of nursing system, per se.[15]

One way in which contemporaries tried to show that the new nursing system was beneficial to the hospitals, the doctors and the patients, was by referring to the length of stay of patients admitted to hospitals; there is some evidence to suggest that there was a general trend towards a reduction in the average length of stay in the voluntary hospitals at the beginning and again at the end of the nineteenth-century. The first reduction was due perhaps to a reorganisation of in-patient facilities rather than any scientific development: the second reduction, according to some historians, may have been due, in part at least, to the way in which the new nurses could be expected and trusted to carry out precisely the orders of superiors, especially doctors. A shorter stay was said to indicate the effectiveness of a treatment regime or its performance by the new nurses: it is more likely, however, that much of the reduction in length of stay was due to an increased demand for bed-usage, particularly at a time when many voluntary hospitals could not open all their wards for lack of funds.[16]

Most writers who comment on the contribution made by nursing to better healthcare provision point out that it was not the trained nurse who actually provided that care at the point of use - the bedside - but the untrained or in-training probationer, whether in a small cottage hospital or 25 beds or a large voluntary hospital of over 700 beds. Contemporaries acknowledged that this was so, although only in official investigations and not in any of the many guides to nursing then available: as White has pointed out, contemporaries "frankly acknowledged that probationer nurses formed the bulk of the nursing staff and that they were 'employed' in preference to trained nurses or nursing attendants since they were the cheapest source of labour. Thus it can be claimed that they subsidised the care of the sick."[17]

If there had been any contribution to improved patient care by nursing in this period it was not through the acquisition by the nurses of 'scientific knowledge' of disease and hygiene, since the holders of that knowledge, the trained nurses did not work at the bedside; the contribution was made through the system of organisation which characterised the new order - a hierarchy of duties and responsibilities together with moral character formation acting through a standardised work routine performed by nurses trained and formed to a standard pattern. In order to understand that contribution we will need to look more closely at those nurses at the bedside, the probationer nurses; we shall need to trace the way in which they came to espouse a common set of nursing values and to perform their tasks aided as well as formed by a characteristic work-discipline; that discussion is taken up in detail in Chapter 2.

The early training schools and definitions of nursing
It would be a mistake to assume that since this study is concerned with the period 1881 - 1914 and deals with the first generation of trained general nurses that nurse training did not exist prior to 1881. Not only were there institutions on the Continent which offered training, usually through bedside experience as opposed to training through formal education, there had been one or two voluntary hospitals in London and in the provinces which had offered some form of training before that date. Perhaps the first English training system of all was given at St. John's House, London, later associated with King's College Hospital, London, started in 1848. The most influential and well-known nurse training was, however, that at the Nightingale School at St. Thomas's Hospital, London, set up in 1860 with the Fund donated by a grateful public in recognition of Florence Nightingale's work in the Crimea.[18]

Nevertheless, these developments did not in themselves provide any significant numbers of nurses, either because they were linked to religious organisations or because the entrants were 'ladies' who merely dabbled philanthropically in nursing as they did in other charitable endeavours, or because the graduates were more concerned to reform hospitals as institutions first and set up training schools for nurses as only a part of that campaign and mission. The first generation of trained general nurses could only be produced once the new order had been implemented in as wide a group of general hospitals as was possible; the first generation were not primarily pioneers or missionaries, nor were they 'nightingales"; they were women who turned to nursing as a choice of work, paid work, rather than one of the many other occupations then available to women, some of which are discussed in the appendix to this chapter.

In the years before 1881 some of these women could have made a reasonable livelihood practising as nurses without any need of evidence of training, although many would have worked for and alongside an older 'nurse' before striking out on their own account. We shall look at the development of the training system and the notion of skill as applied to nursing work later; the mere existence of a formal training and certification was probably sufficient to make more and more women enter a formal nurse training programme after 1881, and the rhetoric of the reformers was perhaps not as necessary as they and subsequent writers assumed.

Before the Nurse Registration Act (1919) there was no legal definition of a nurse: even after the Act the only nurse defined by law was a State Registered Nurse, one who had been registered by the General Nursing Council. Even after 1919 it was in order for a woman or man to call her/himself a nurse provided that the impression was not given that 'nurse' meant State Registered.[19]

The word nurse derives, via Old French, from the Latin 'nutricius' meaning nourishing;[20] this was not just a semantic exercise for contemporaries, it was of vital importance to those anxious to establish hospital nursing as the superior form of the occupation. While a nurse-in-health role, like that performed by Juliet's companion or duenna, was consistent with Nightingale's broad theory of nursing, one definition of which included "the nursing the sick and injured, Preventative or Sanitary Nursing, or nursing healthy children",[21] most reformers found it convenient to forget the notion that all women were nurses. In place of the aphorism "every woman is a nurse", contemporaries substituted the idea that all women could be taught to nurse.

It was acknowledged by many that while women were born with a predisposition for specific social roles, these innate qualities could only flourish through education and training. No woman could expect to automatically become a good wife, mother or even 'lady'; in the complex society of late-Victorian England women needed help to draw out their natural attributes in order to make the most effective use of them. That educative process was set first of all in the family home, where the mother by her own example, and the father by his strict adherence to a moral discipline, helped the girl to develop into a good woman. In order to help in this process, manuals of home-management and courses in domestic science were produced and made widely available; while this contemporary concern with the training of women was geared towards marriage, or towards the already married woman trying to better herself as a home-manager, it also carried over into the debate about nurse training. It was not that women were not by nature nurses, rather it was necessary for women to learn more about the complexities of nursing, the science of nursing, in order to be more effective at their natural duties as daughters, wives and sisters.[22]

Since more people were going into hospitals to be cared for, thus usurping part of the role of the woman in the family, the women who looked after hospital patients had to be shown how to do so most efficiently. Even if the middle-classes were not entering hospitals in large numbers, preferring to be cared for in their own homes, the complex nature of disease and its modern treatment regimes required the women who nursed them to also have some training in the new science of nursing.

Perhaps a more important cause for the shift in emphasis in nursing was the contemporary realisation that nursing was becoming another area of work for all women, and not just the widowed and the religious. In part this had come as one of the consequences of the demographic changes noted in mid-century, loosely termed 'the surplus woman problem';[23] new work opportunities were sought by an increasing section of unsupported females particularly from the middle-classes. It was also due to the influence of the early middle-class women who went into nursing in order to reform it, women like Agnes Jones, Elizabeth Fry and Nightingale herself: according to some commentators, their early involvement with nursing had helped to give it the aura not of respectability but of missionary zeal leading towards respectability. Nursing had also become an area of work opportunity for women from late century onwards as a direct consequence of the structural changes in the economy; we shall look at the changing work opportunities for women below; here we may note that nursing was only one of many "white-blouse" jobs being opened up in the late-nineteenth- and early-twentieth-centuries.

Whatever the explanations for the shift in the construct of every-woman as nurse to every-woman may be trained to nurse, training for nursing and the method by which that training should be measured became of central importance to the occupation after the 1880's, culminating in the movement for the State Registration of nurses. Definitions of what constituted a nurse became important as areas of dispute within the occupation, although all factions were agreed on one crucial element making up a nurse - her distinction from a doctor in gender, knowledge and practice.[24]

The contemporary confusion, both within the occupation and in the public arena, was used by some reformers, like the Fenwicks,[25] to strengthen their case for a closed profession. The Select Committee on the Registration of Nurses (1905) was presented with a list of 89 "typical nursing scandals" taken from newspapers by the Fenwicks to prove that women of ques-

tionable moral character were duping an unsuspecting public as
to their 'professional' status as nurses.[26] Among the cases
they cited were abortionists, thieves and prostitutes, all of
who appeared to have called themselves nurses either to carry
out their 'crimes' or to gain sympathy from the courts when
they were tried. Despite the fact that many of the "typical
scandals" were found not guilty, and despite the Select Committee's feeling that their existence did not prejudice the
public's estimation of the professional nurse, the Fenwicks
made much capital in their campaign for registration out of
the mere suggestion that such scandals might take place. The
public, they argued, had the right to know what a nurse was,
what duties and responsibilities she had in the sickroom, what
measure of trust could the family of an ill-person place in
her; a woman wishing to earn her living as a nurse, they demanded, had to be a trained nurse.[27]

Two features were to mark the new general nurse as different not only from the old gamps but as different from other
types of nurses in the modern period: first, she was technically trained and up to date with contemporary medical practice; second, she was a trained woman, with all that that implied in terms of character, subordination and purpose. Technical expertise, even if it meant a little more than "taking
the patient's temperature and pulse correctly and ... accurately reporting ... to the doctor" which Dr. Bedford
Fenwick had said it did,[28] could be instilled through a formal system of education, through lectures, demonstrations and
examinations. The development of the qualities of womanhood in
the nurse was not so easily achieved, not least because the
first hurdle which had to be overcome was the idea that all
women could nurse automatically. To bring out the true woman
as nurse, the training system had to instil a rigid code of
behaviour and self-discipline in the woman, to top up any
quality deficient in the entrant or to draw out to the maxi-
mum the natural talent of the woman.[29]

The process of moral training, which emphasised above all
the quality of obedience, was largely an informal process, a
code of behaviour which the recruit learnt in the same way as
a child, by making mistakes and being punished, by doing well
and being rewarded. The home motif, the family imagery, which
percolated this hospital discipline was based on the middle-
class construct of the family with its division of roles and
spheres, rights and duties, and clear distinctions between the
sexes. In the hospital world the doctors assumed the role of
the father and in his absence (since he had little to do with
nurses anyway) the functions of the father were subsumed under
the functions of the mother, the senior nurse. Obeying the
senior nurses, ward sisters, nurse-tutors, matrons as well as
Home Sisters, meant that the trainee was obeying the doctor/
father: in the event, accepting and maintaining the divisions
of labour between grades of trainees - standing up in the pre-

sence of a nurse only months the senior, allowing them to pass
through the door before you, even making the life on the on-
trial probationer in her first days difficult, could all be
explained and justified by reference to this clear acknowledgement of the authority of the doctor/man.

So strong was the imagery of the family that some commentators, faced with the obvious fact that more and more women
were not fulfilling their 'true natures' through marriage and
family life, made conscious efforts to extend the construct of
the family to encompass humanity itself. In this way Saleeby,
an eugenicist and a doctor, encouraged women to take up nursing instead of trying, futilely perhaps, to find a husband -

> It is not necessarily argued, by any means, that mar-
> riage and motherhood are to be set forth as the goals
> at which every girl is to aim; such a woman as Miss
> Florence Nightingale was a Foster-Mother to countless
> thousands, and was only the greatest exemplar in our
> time of a function which is essentially womanly, but
> does not involve marriage." (original emphasis).[30]

- nurses, therefore, were the 'mothers' of the poor, the sick
and, indeed, the world.

The prescriptive model of the new nurse
The expanding hospital and non-institutional healthcare sectors needed a larger labour force than that which the existing
nursing population could provide. The hospitals, therefore, set
about recruiting women to nursing, and in particular to nurse
training since such novices could be expected to take on the
new methods more readily than nurses used to working on their
own account or under the lax system which had characterised the
old hospital regimes. Trainees were also preferred because they
were the cheapest form of labour for hospitals which faced the
constant problems of under-financing, whether they were voluntary supported or publically supported through the rates. That
recruitment, however, took place in the context of structural
changes in the economy which resulted in changes in work opportunities for women in particular (see Appendix, below). As a
consequence of the service revolution and the growth of "white-
blouse" work,[31] nursing had to compete for recruits with other
occupations; nursing had to offer those who took it up something in exchange for the harsh conditions of service, long
hours, lack of personal control over day-to-day living, and so
on.[32] As we shall see, nursing had to offer some explanation
for "menial work", like cleaning lavatories and spittoons,
which went beyond the need to keep the wards clean (since domestic servants could do that just as easily as a nurse).

The first, or perhaps the last, thing which general nursing offered the woman considering nursing as a career was
status, the public and occupational acknowledgement of a special role in the care of the sick which was denied to other

14

workers. The hospital-trained general nurse was to be the epitome of the new nursing order, her reliability, honesty, sobriety, diligence and punctuality reflections of the system which created her, and a direct and obvious contrast with the Gamps and the Prigs she supplanted. That that process was being worked through during our period is evidenced by the contemporary concern with registration and with making the occupation a closed one:[33] in practical terms that superiority was shown by the way in which the general nurse was able to obtain senior posts in nursing and allied fields by virtue of the initial general training alone.

While the promise of a future to come may have persuaded some women into the work, such farsightedness cannot have been so commonplace a feature of contemporary adolescence and early adulthood to explain why so many women did take up the work. Nursing had to offer, therefore, something equivalent to the status of the trained nurse - exclusivity - but at the earlier stage, in training; that reward was to be one of a select group of women with special characteristics, who were somehow 'ordained' to become nurses. We need, then, to look at the image generated by the occupation of the ideal recruit and the nurse-in-training; there we shall see the immediacy of the reward for undertaking the dedication of service to humanity and the acceptance of the rigorous life of the nurse-in-training.

We can identify certain core features making up the composite ideal recruit and nurse-in-training; first, the age at which women chose nursing; second, the previous work experiences of the entrant to nursing; third, the educational background of the recruit and fourth, the social origins of the recruits which may have predisposed them to take up nursing.[34] To a greater or lesser extent, all of the contemporary 'theoretical' discussions about the type of recruit needed under the new nursing order included a statement relating to each of these elements, and while there were differences - for example, some reformers thought nursing training could begin at 23, others not until 25 years of age - all felt that these were important determining factors in the make-up of the ideal recruit.

According to all commentators, the relatively high age of entry, about 23 years in the voluntary hospitals and 21 in the Poor Law hospitals in 1908, was determined by the physically - and mentally - demanding nature of caring for the sick and the dying. Writing in a textbook for nurses issued in 1901, Voysey told the potential nurse

> No-one ought to think of training before twenty-one years of age - 25 is better ... The work is very arduous, and no-one, except those who have been through training, has any idea of how trying it can be and what a strain is put upon the mind and body. It should be seriously considered how far that body can bear the strain, unless it be immaterial to become a total wreck

- a disaster which is not at all uncommon, and which
may easily happen if the constitution is not very
good, or has a history of weakness.[35]

Most contemporary nurse-writers seem to have been agreed
that full physical and mental development was attained by the
women only after the age of twenty-one and that twenty-five
was the optimum age for training.[36] Even when the minimum age
for entry was reduced c1910, (when it became apparent that
there were insufficient women aged 25-plus willing to enter
nursing), writers still cautioned the intending nurse to wait
until she was at least twenty-three.[37] Arguing that the reduction in the recommended age of entry was due to the "better
conditions" of service for recruits and nurses in the first
decades of the twentieth-century, (and not perhaps the desperate need for recuits of any age), many nurse-writers suggested that only at those hospitals which themselves cared for
their nurses was the physical and mental harshness of training
recognised;[38] a hospital offering training to any woman under
23 (or perhaps 21) years of age was not a "hospital of repute",
and was only interested in meeting the needs of filling its
wards with 'nurses' of any standard.[39]
As well as a minimum age of entry, most contemporaries
warned of the dangers of turning to nursing too late in life;
the very hard life of a nurse, which threatened to wreck the
health of the under-twenty-three year old, could also destroy
the woman aged over thirty-five. Such older entrants would
"find the training a heavy tax on both their mental and physical strength", especially the long hours of night-duty which
was required of all nurses before being granted a certificate.
[40] One problem which the older recruit faced and which the
younger did not, apparently, was the slowing down of her mental faculties, her reluctance to change from which had perhaps
become the entrenched habits of a lifetime. The woman over
thirty-five had "usually lost adaptability and the powers of
readily receiving new impressions", and she would find the
necessity for study and for learning the science of nursing
more difficult because of her age.[41] More importantly, however,
at least as far as the qualified older nurse was concerned, she
would have to compete for the new senior nursing posts with
women trained to the same standard but much younger and thus
more adaptable and willing to work harder and longer in order
to transform nursing itself through their example and their
authority.[42]
The suggestion that there was an ideal age at which to
begin training was justified in the literature by reference to
the hard work which was nursing and by arguing that the new
generation of trained general nurses would have to work harder
not only because they were representatives of the new order,
but also because by working harder they could help to get rid
of the old style nurse, characterised so frequently as the

inactive Sairey Gamp or Betsy Prig. The experiences of many matrons also bore out this determination to recruit from an age range between 23 and 30, since they knew that many of the trainees who left the occupation did so because of ill-health brought on by nursing, or exaccerbated by the conditions under which so many nurses worked.

The age-bar, while not official nor necessarily an attempt to restrict entry to an ideal type, was perhaps an early attempt to reduce the casualty rate especially during training. However, the promulgation of a preferred age of entry to training had inferences beyond the overt desire to enrol healthy recruits; the age range which nursing literature put forward as most desirable was closely linked to the age range at which women were most likely to face the work/marriage decision stage in their life. Nurses were, therefore, being asked to choose between marriage and a career; whether that choice was real or not was immaterial; the importance lay in the apparent choice and those who perhaps chose nursing rather than marriage could be described as having opted for the service of mankind rather than of a man.[43]

Putting forward a minimum age of entry left nursing reformers with a gap in the pre-training picture of the nurse-recruit's life; what did the ideal trainee do between leaving school and starting nurse training 7 or 8 years later? At first the ideal recruit was firmly placed within the bosom of her family, at her mother's side and under her instruction:

> A knowledge of housework is essential. It was a wise matron who told an intending probationer to go home and be her mother's housemaid for six months, and then apply to her again. Cleanliness is the first thing taught in nursing. The nurse should be a teacher of hygiene in all its branches, and how can she do this if she does not herself lead the way?[44]

Another writer lamented the 'modern' girl's eagerness to leave the family home too soon - "it seems almost a pity that these early days in a girl's life should be subject to hospital restrictions and that she should lack the home care so necessary for her when she first leaves school" - and she advised those girls thinking of taking up nursing to wait until the general hospitals were willing to take her, at the best age, i.e. 23 years.[45]

It was this development, that girls were seeking to nurse too early, which forced many writers to acknowledge this 'natural urge' to spread their wings and enter the world of work, and to care for others. Many writers of nursing guides after the turn of the century devoted at least a paragraph or two to the advantages and disadvantages of work, and nursing work, before entry to general training. A few continued to suggest that the true nurse would not engage in any sort of work before training, while some modified this extreme position by suggesting that if the girl really wanted to do something 'useful' before nursing, she should undertake some form of charitable and unpaid work, which in the closing decades of the nineteenth- and opening years of the twentieth-centuries had burgeoned.

Others, perhaps more aware of the contemporary changes in work opportunities for women as well as the need most girls had to work anyway, tried to indicate certain types of work which the intending general nurse could fairly safely take up in the years before entry to training. Usually such jobs were linked to household functions, and more often than not included the opportunity for some degree of instruction or training which could then prove useful to the nurse in her later career.[46] Girls who had to work, out of an intense longing to 'do something' or out of necessity - "if a girl is compelled to either partially or wholly support herself as soon as her education is finished" - were advised to "choose an occupation of such a kind that she will be equiping herself directly and indirectly for her future life."[47] While few examples of actual work experiences which would fit this plan were ever offered, potential recruits to general nurse training were warned to choose "some definite business"

> where there are regular duties to fulfil, regular hours to keep, and where neatness, method, quickness and punctuality are necessary. The one thing she should not do during these years is to dawdle about at home idly amusing herself, and letting others wait upon her and do all the real work of the house. A girl can be placed in no circumstances in which she cannot cultivate the virtues, so essential in hospitals, of helpfulness, patience, quickness, tact and neatness. The fewer bad habits she has to eradicate in the wards the more time she will find for learning what can only be taught there; and she can learn at home quite as well as anywhere else how to walk about an uncarpeted floor quietly, how to keep a room neat and clean, and how to shut a door securely without banging it.[48]

With hardly an exception, all writers advising girls on pre-nursing work were at pains to point out the pitfalls inherent in taking a preliminary nursing qualification, such as fever or mental training.[49] Part of their disapproval centred on the consequent total time the girl would spend in-training if she then went on to become a general nurse; time spent in training, as we have noted, was said to be the hardest part of the nurse's life, both mentally and physically, and these advisors were concerned to reduce the drop-out rate among such women. It also delayed the time when the girl would be a trained nurse in her own right, and hence could train others and take part in the missionary duty which Nightingale-inspired rhetoric had mapped out for her.[50]

A more strongly argued case against pre-general nursing experience and training was the problem which the 'nurse' would face when she came to take general training. While many acknowledged that "knowledge of any kind is valuable" and an understanding of hospital routine and discipline would prevent many such women committing the faux-pas which might "prejudice their teachers against them" during general training, most warned the girl thinking of an early entry to nursing via one of the specialist branches that

> All matrons do not care for probationers who have
> had preliminary training: they think, perhaps, the
> partially trained nurse is more difficult to train
> than the novice ... and that, however much know-
> ledge she may have acquired elsewhere, her rank on
> starting to train will be that only of a junior pro-
> bationer, and as such she must behave.[51]

Women were not advised, then, to take up nursing in the small hospitals or in the specialised areas of nursing, even if they offered a training and a certificate of competence: extending the in-training period from three or four years to perhaps six or seven years would only lead to an even earlier physical (or mental) breakdown than might be expected. The apparent status which the specialist nurse had because of her early training would have to be given up when she entered the general hospital and some of these women might resent having to become very junior probationers again. Such 'trained' nurses might not readily accept the need for a return to the rigid discipline of the probationer's existence in the general hospitals, and, as many writers pointed out, the standards of discipline expected of the general nurse in training were far higher than those in the specialist or smaller hospitals. The traumatic experience of becoming a probationer after being a trained nurse could lead many such women to give up general training and even give up nursing altogether: the general matrons and their propagandists were, therefore, only acting in the best interests of the women in advising them not to undertake any nursing, whether it offered training or not, before entering general nurse training itself.

However, such advice was not without its consequences, intended or not; by telling women that they should not work before nursing, or at least only work in areas useful to their futures as nurses, the writers of such guides were showing the pre-nursing experiences as only a temporary phase in the women's life. They thus set out to prevent women interested in becoming nurses finding themselves other careers in which they might then wish to remain, or to prevent them from entering

nursing too early and in the wrong field, finding out that
they did not like it, and were thus lost to the occupation entirely. While some women, as we shall see, left nursing quite
early on in their training because they discovered it was not
for them, general nursing felt it could reduce that leaving
rate by offering the entrant an alternative reason or set of
reasons for remaining in training and for becoming a general
nurse, that is, exclusiveness and status. The argument, then,
was somewhat circular; status was ascribed to the entrant to
general training by virtue of that training, which could only
be undertaken by certain 'special' women, some of whom were
special because they did not choose to enter any of the other
branches of nursing first. As we shall discuss in Chapter 2,
this set of advice to intending nurses appears either to have
been ignored or else to have been adapted to suit the realities of the recruitment policies, or indeed the realities of
most women's lives.

The recommended age of entry to general nurse training
and the way in which the intending nurse was advised to spend
the waiting years were linked not only in the way in which
such advice argued for a special status for general nursing
but also by the idea that in those years the woman would be
acquiring skills and knowledge which would be helpful in her
later career as a nurse. It was assumed that any education
received in that time was 'higher' education, and not the acquisition of the basic skills taught in the schools of the
period. However, at a time when compulsory education at elementary and secondary level was only being introduced gradually, especially education beyond the age of 13 years, it is
difficult to know what contemporary nurse leaders considered
to be a good basic education for the intending probationer.

Rarely did any contemporary define what was meant by a
good educational standard for training, although all hospitals
insisted that the applicants for training be educated to that
level. In 1898, Chelsea Poor Law Infirmary required "a fair
education" of the applicants, while Manchester Royal Infirmary
expected recruits to be "well educated".[52] Voysey, speaking
for many matrons, said that the intending probationer "should
be able to read and write clearly and have sufficient mental
capacity for understanding the study of medical and surgical
cases from the doctors' point of view, not that she might
criticise, but intelligently receive his instructions and
carry out his orders".[53]

The educational standard required of the recruit was,
therefore, linked to the formal training needs and to the
carrying out of routine tasks on the wards at the doctors'
instruction, albeit through the person of the ward sister.
Since contemporary education varied considerably both region-
ally and by social group, many hospitals set some form of test
of educational achievement before allowing women to proceed to
full training. That test might be simply the filling in of an

application form for a post, "in the candidate's own hand"; it might be a written test during the interview with the matron for a place in the training hospital, or it might form the test taken at the end of the trial period prior to signing the training contract and entering general nurse training proper. Such tests, usually of general knowledge, helped to weed out those who might not be able to read treatment charts or instructions,[54] or the nursing textbooks used during the course of instruction in the training programme; they also served to enhance the apparent difficulty of gaining entrance to the occupation and hence the prestige of being accepted for training. Only in rare exceptions was some form of entrance test of educational standard waived, and only then if the applicant could provide "acceptable evidence of equivalent examination"; [55] this juxtaposition of the entrance-to-nursing test and other examinations, perhaps of recognised state education bodies, served to further represent the nursing test as a difficult hurdle to be overcome only by 'educated' women.

Perhaps the only women who might automatically claim exemption from the entrance test were those women entering nursing from the middle-classes, women who could be expected to have been educated to a high level. While the education of middle-class women still lagged behind that of middle-class men, in standard as well as in content, developments since mid-century had worked to ensure that fewer middle-class women were prevented from acquiring often a wide range of educational knowledge by their late teens.[56] Whether that education was acquired by attendance at one of the growing number of schools for such girls, or by being taught by a governess or tutor, middle-class women were, by the turn of the century, no less exposed to formal education than middle-class men or even working-class children.

The existence of a small core of middle-class entrants, both as pioneers in the earlier decades and as 'ordinary' entrants towards the end of our period, women with a considerable standard of education who would not have to sit any entrance test, meant that those entrants who passed an 'equivalent' test, i.e. the nursing entrance examination, and who were not middle-class, could consider themselves, educationally at least, equivalent to these middle-class women. Successful entrants could take on some of the prestige attached to being middle-class by virtue of a common standard of education.

That core of middle-class nurses, while as important in nursing as in other women's occupations in the nineteenth-century in terms of status and habits of gentility etc.,[57] were numerically insignificant, as contemporaries themselves acknowledged.[58] As we shall discuss in the Chapter dealing with the recruitment to general nurse training, the class from which recruits were drawn was seen by many to be an important question for the status and future of nursing itself. While many acknowledged the debt owed to the middle-class and even lower aristocratic entrants and pioneers, most nurse commentators knew the occupation to be at least "mixed as to rank", if not absolutely composed of women from the 'lower orders';[59] however, even when admitting this, the nurses did not speak of women from the working-class in general, but women from an "earnest class";[60] it would seem that such women could be found in all walks of life, working- and middle-class, and indeed their earnestness was what wiped out the social distinctions of class of which contemporaries were acutely aware. Even if they were aware of the differences between the types of women found in the training, the standard form of instruction and the standardisation of the training programme itself would wipe out any vestiges of 'class', and turn all women into trained nurses and thus members of the earnest class.

While contemporaries were rightly keen to recruit those who could read and write and study under guidance, their lack of clarity about what constituted a good standard of education was made up for by their certainty about the type of woman required. Class origin and social background were less important than the possession of certain basic virtues, including obedience, truthfulness and kindheartedness; these characteristics were those ascribed to good women in general, rather than women belonging to one or other social class.[61]

Nowhere was the decisiveness about the sort of woman needed by nursing more plainly stated, nor with such force, as in the many debates about the type of tasks which nurses had to perform, and in particular those which were termed "menial" and have since become known as 'non-nursing duties'.

The 'problem' owes its origin almost inevitably to Nightingale herself; while she saw the cleaning of the room, of the environment of sickness and health, as proper work for the nurse, she failed to make it clear to her followers when such tasks should be carried out by the nurse herself and when they might satisfactorily be left to a lower grade of worker supervised by the trained nurse:[62] in part this was the consequence of the contemporary state of hospitals and wards and the need she felt to raise the standard of public hygiene quickly; in part it was also a reluctance to intrude on what she perceived as the territory and responsibility of the medical profession.[63]

Even at St. Thomas' Hospital after her intervention, Nightingale insisted on keeping on the 'old' nurses alongside of, or rather some way beneath, the new nurses in training; these women were to actually carry out the instructions of the 'nightingales', relieving them of every menial duty and freeing them for instruction by the sister and the matron and, of course, the doctors.[64] A hierarchy of authority and duties thus emerged in the new order, which was transferred (and suffered transcription in the process) to other hospitals; at the apex was the trained general nurse, at the base the ward scrubber or the newly engaged junior probationer, depending on the individual hospital's system.

The newly entered probationer was therefore faced with the prospect of performing tasks which she might not have associated with modern nursing, such as cleaning lavatories, washbasins, inkstands, sputum-pots, or bedsteads. The entrant had to be shown that the performance of such tasks was vital not only to the new order of nursing, via the science of hygiene, but to herself as a representative of that order. Cleaning, domestic, or menial tasks were therefore performed because they were part of the science of nursing, asepsis and antisepsis, or were part of the characteristics of the new nurse.

Opposition to performing such tasks came both from within the occupation and from outside; in 1893 one probationer wrote to the Manchester local paper complaining of the menial work performed by the probationers at the Royal Infirmary; she said

> the probationers or day nurses should not be required to scour the floors of the wards, the cupboards and other menial work of that kind which they at present have to do ... [65]

In the same year, the authoress and social commentator, Mrs. Ormiston Chant had written in a nursing journal that probationers and other grades of nurses should not have to do domestic work because it gave them such rough hands, causing acute discomfort to their patients.[66] A more systematic attack on domestic duties performed by nurses came in a series of articles written by Lady Priestly which appeared in <u>Nineteenth Century</u> (1897), in which she sought to question many of the nursing reformers' claims about the better status of the new nurses.[67]

Counter-attacks came from within the occupation; Nightingale herself attempted to repair some of the damage done by her original remarks, but perhaps only added to the problem:

> If a nurse declines to do certain things for her patient 'because it is not her business', I should say that nursing was not her calling. I have seen surgical 'sisters' down on their knees scouring a room or hut, because they thought it otherwise not fit for their patients to go into. I am far from wishing nurses to scour. It is a waste of power. (sic) But I do say that these women had the true nurse-calling - the good of their sick first, and second only the consideration of what is their 'place' to do - and that women who wait for the housemaid to do this, or for the charwoman to do that, when their patients are suffering, have not the <u>making</u> of a nurse in them.
> (original emphasis)[68]

In reply to the letter from the Manchester probationer, cited above, a "nurse-sympathiser" wrote "training, in the sense which nurses require it embraces habits of order, cleanliness, gentleness, and quietness, without these the theoretical training would be worth nothing and no true woman would object to scouring provided it is for the good of the patients." (emphasis added).[69]

By the turn of the century, when the general trained nurse was a common-place feature of hospital and nursing worlds, the idea that the true nurse was a true woman who did all the menial tasks necessary for the care of her patient had become translated into the idea that the professional general trained nurse did such tasks because she was a good woman and a trained nurse. From about 1900 onwards the debate broadened out into a discussion of which grade of personnel should do which grade of 'menial' work, although as one writer pointed out, "the word menial does not properly enter the trained nurses' vocabulary".[70] The seminal discussion about what properly constituted nursing as opposed to non-nursing menial work was provided by the anonymous "Late Matron" in The Hospital (1901). The term menial work as applied to nursing had become "ward work" in this article, and in it the matron asked what ward work meant; to her it was

> all those duties, the performance of which is essential to the good environment of patients, but which in themselves form no part of medical treatment, or nursing, in strict terms, i.e., sweeping, dusting, polishing or scrubbing of floors etc. ... In some hospitals a large part of a probationer's time is taken up with domestic duties - sweeping, scrubbing of floors, lockers, tables, baths, crockery, polishing of innumerable brass taps, cleaning of sinks, washing of glass globes, etc. In another institution some only of these tasks are expected of a nurse.[71]

The line between the proper duties of the nurse and those of her inferiors, ward cleaners and scrubbers, was to be drawn between those duties which had "close connections with nursing", those tasks which referred for their rationale to the science of hygiene and public health, and those which were linked to the cleaning of the institution, general housework.[72]

However, there was not only a hierarchy of tasks as between nurse and wardmaid: there was also a distinction between the ward work performed by the trained nurse and that performed by the junior, since only those women who had had training, even if it was only six months more than the raw recruit, had access to the science of nursing. The very junior probationer, then, could be and was left with all of the domestic duties which her particular hospital chose to delegate to the nursing staff rather than employ wardmaids.

In creating this hierarchy it was argued that the new entrant would learn to better accept the hospital discipline, to appreciate the value of her training and learn how to manage others who would be her subordinates in the future, once more reiterating and reinforcing the Nightingale-dictum that the trained nurse was trained to train, rather than to nurse.[73] Control of others, be they patients, wardmaids or nurses-in-training, was the major role of the new trained nurse, but before she could control others by virtue of her training, she had to learn to control herself through that training: as Nightingale had warned some probationers in training at St. Thomas's, "the very first element for having control over others is, of course, to have control over oneself. If I cannot take charge of myself, I cannot take charge of others".[74]

Because control in this sense was equated with moral character, and since the training of the new nurse involved this crucial component, tasks which appeared to be non-nursing duties could be used to inculcate self-discipline, to help the trainees learn how to control others by learning to control themselves. Just as the girl wanting to know how to spend the time between school and nurse training had been advised to learn at her mother's side the management of a home, so the girl who had not benefitted from such an opportunity or for some reason had not been given that opportunity, could still learn that element, (which was also described as unquestioning obedience to superiors). by accepting without dispute the necessity of performing duties she did not immediately see as her proper sphere. One matron reiterated the value of wardwork for the nurse-in-training;

> to repeat the question, 'why should ward work form part of a nurse's training?' That she may know how to instruct those who are suitable by up-bringing and the accident of birth for such work. This satisfies common sense, and should be inducement enough to a nurse to acquire during a short time of her probationership a thorough knowledge of a wardmaid's duties, as embraced by 'ward work'. All those who have held authority know that to direct and supervise the work of others is a far stricter discipline than the performance of that work oneself ...[75]

Thus, the nurse who had been through the training of a general nurse could be a manager of others, patients or nurses, precisely because she had herself had experience of all of the tasks she asked her subordinates to perform, even though that experience might have been for a very short time indeed. What allowed her to claim superiority despite only a short experience of such tasks was not only that experience but her training in the rationale for such duties; her train-

ing in self-control accompanied her training in the science
of nursing, and she not only knew how to do these duties but
why they had to be carried out efficiently. The general
trained nurse was, then, not only a maid-of-all-work, but the
mistress of all.

'Occupational imperialism': The supremacy of the general nurse
As we have noted, the education of the general nurse worked to
produce not only the technically competent and confident nurse,
but also a nurse who saw herself as a member of an elite group
because of her training; the details of that process will be
examined in the following chapters. However, the idea of
superiority which the general trained nurse felt was not expressed solely in her own sphere, the general hospitals, and
over just patients and junior nurses. If the general nurse was
to really reign supreme, she had to demonstrate her elite status outside of her immediate area; the general trained nurse
had to take over other areas of nursing and extend her control
of others to include specialist nurses and other healthcare
workers, and in this period this in essence meant the doctors.
     Chapter 4 of this study deals in some detail with the way
in which general nurses moved out of their training hospitals
and into other areas of nursing, usually at senior levels,
thus displacing incumbent specialists, which in turn acted to
encourage such nurses to turn to general training themselves
in order to compete with this development.
     The extension of the general nurse's control over others
to include other members of the healthcare workforce was not
so easily accomplished. As the nurses in training had learnt,
the doctor directed and the nurse obeyed, intelligently perhaps, but undoubtedly unquestionably. How, then, could the
general nurse exert any form of control over this group, who
were not only her occupational superiors but were also men,
and hence to be obeyed on two counts?
     For those general trained nurses who went into private
practice the opportunity for exerting or demonstrating this
superiority over doctors lay in their new technical expertise.
The sort of doctor they could expect to have to deal with was
the general practitioner, members of that group of doctors who
had evolved largely from the apothecary system of English medicine.[76] Such doctors, with exceptions, prided themselves on
their autonomy from the consultant system within the hospital
medical schools, which was shown in their reluctance to call
in such consultants in their cases and in the internal dis-
putes which had bedevilled the registration of medical practitioners.[77] These general practitioners were faced with competition for their services from the hospital network, voluntary and Poor Law, or if that competition was not so direct,
at least from the difficulties many experienced in actually
finding and building up a general practice of their own.[78]
     The appearance of another group of workers who might

cream off some of their hard-won patients, i.e. the new general nurses, was a real fear for many general practitioners and opposition to the very idea of nurse training by the medical profession came most vehemently from this group. Some argued along traditional lines of attack, linking nursing and its horrors with the degradation of femininity;[79] most developed their attack along the lines that competition for patients would have disastrous consequences for an unsuspecting public.[80]

Similar attacks had been successfully used to criticise the existence of female midwives and although that campaign had actually resulted in the State regulation of midwives (1902) it had also had the effect of severely limiting the ability of women to work as midwives, thus transferring that area of income and practice to the effective control of doctors and of men.[81]

In the specialist hospitals, and indeed the Poor Law hospitals when they were 'invaded' by the voluntary hospital trained nurses, the automatic authority of the doctor over the management of the institution was not clearly defined. Either this was because the hospital was run by a Board of Guardians as in the case of the Poor Law infirmaries, the fever hospitals, sanatoria and mental asylums, where the doctor was but another employee of the institution, or else the specialist institution had so few doctors constantly on the premises as to leave a gap through which the new general nurse could drive her personality and her superiority. In such cases, the organisational skills which she had been taught as a general nurse, rather than her technical competence, were her main weapons in establishing her influence.[82]

Such developments were not unopposed, of course, nor did they last particularly long once the medical profession realised what was happening (or indeed, once the lay administrators themselves came to flex their considerable organisational muscle), but the missionary zeal which frequently accompanied the entry of the general nurse into such areas comforted the new nurse when she was faced with opposition to her rule. Indeed, she knew she could always leave that institution, leave it to its fate, as so many of the original nightingales had done, deciding that such institutions were not ready or fit to be brought into the new order.[83]

Whether real or apparent, the notion that the trained general nurse could go anywhere in the world of nursing, and literally anywhere in the world, played an important part not only in helping to produce the confident superior general nurse but in convincing the recipients of her attentions of the supremacy of her skills. That process we might usefully describe as 'occupational imperialism', a metaphor which includes in it the idea of bringing progress to underdeveloped or backward areas, and of instructing those areas in the means of self-development but not in the means of self-determination:

it is also an apposite description of the function which medical care and hence the new order of nursing played in contemporary society. As one critical commentator argued, the new hospitals and the new order of medical and nursing care in them were needed not only to check and cure diseases, "but because they mitigate the sufferings of the poor, and tend to produce peace and harmony between the different classes of society."

> The evils which the dangers of the present political
> and social state of the world threaten to bring
> about, can be mitigated socially and physically by
> no other institutions better than a system of well-
> provided voluntary hospitals.[84]

Sources and structure of the study

This study has made use of the usual sources available to historians, including Parliamentary Papers, contemporary books and articles, and the mass of secondary works relevant to its theme. However, it has been necessary to look for other data and sources specific to a study of the experiences of the rank and file member of an occupation, since most of the available sources confine themselves to the leadership of that occupation or to views about the 'ordinary' worker by the leadership. If we are to understand how the individual general trained nurse came to be trained and to take part in the process we have called occupational imperialism, we need to get as close to her as possible, even if that involves us in re-evaluating existing data in the light of new questions.[85]

Three major sources have been added to the more usual catalogue for this present study of nursing, as well as the reworking of more traditional sources; original hospital records; oral evidence, and fiction represented mainly in the novels of the period. Before looking in detail at the data in the following chapters, it will be necessary to briefly examine these sources and their relevance to the present study of nursing 1881 - 1914.

An attempt has been made to select data from a range of hospitals, metropolitan and provincial, Poor Law and voluntary: in part this was a deliberate attempt to counteract the London-orientated bias within existing accounts of nursing, to extend the discussion of the development of general nursing to the many local hospitals which, while acknowledging the importance of the London hospitals in determining nursing policies, had local criteria in mind when developing their own nurse training schemes.

Since many hospitals have not kept material which could be useful in a study such as this, the sample was somewhat determined by the availability of records. The major records used here are the hospital records, Letter Books, Minutes of various Committees, Matron's Reports and Employee Registers,

found at the following hospitals: Manchester Royal Infirmary:
Leeds Poor Law Infirmary; The London Hospital; Southampton
Poor Law Infirmary; Portsmouth Poor Law Infirmary; the Royal
South Hants Infirmary, Southampton; the Royal Hants Infirmary,
Winchester; Salisbury General Infirmary, and the Poplar and
Stepney Poor Law Asylum.

Not all hospitals used here provide the same type or
amount of material, nor frequently for truly comparable
periods, especially those records relating to nurses in training; indeed, this run of data was largely determined by the
date at which each hospital began formal probationer training.
[86] Broadly speaking, records concerning probationers are
available from

1857	Royal South Hants Infirmary
1881	The London Hospital
1881	Manchester Royal Infirmary
1895	Leeds Poor Law Infirmary
1895	Royal Hants Infirmary
1895	Poplar and Stepney Asylum
1896	Salisbury General Infirmary
1902	Southampton Poor Law Infirmary
1905	Portsmouth Poor Law Infirmary

The insights and personalities which some of the hospital
records occasionally reveal, (since few were written in the
expectation of being read by anyone other than the matron or
her successors), are available to the historian from another
source, the personal witness. There are, throughout this study,
references to personal experiences of nurses, found usually in
autobiographies written at the end of the nurse's career.[87]
One disadvantage of such accounts is that the witness cannot
be questioned, to explain more fully an observation or to
raise topics not dealt with by that author. Interviewing the
witness in person overcomes some of these drawbacks, and the
use of the tape- and film-recorder allows more time for more
questions to be posed. In the present study some use has been
made of oral testimony, obtained by means of a small scale
oral history project carried out by the author between 1977 -
1980.

Since the literature is by now well established,[88] this
is not the place to debate the advantages and disadvantages of
obtaining data by such a method; indeed, even those historians
opposed to the idea that there is such a discipline as 'oral
history' acknowledge that many of them use the personal interview as an important means of checking information or queries
raised from other sources. This, for example, is the stance
taken by many political historians, for example A.J.P. Taylor,
who admitted that he often used the friendly fireside chat to
check on his data.[89]

In this study, the small scale nature of the sample can-

not attempt to provide anything like the mass of evidence collected by such large scale projects as that of Paul Thompson
and Thea Vigne at the University of Essex;[90] however, the data
from even a small scale oral evidence project "serves as a
measure of authenticity, a forcible reminder that the historian's categories must in the end correspond to the grain of
human experience, and be constituted from it, if they are to
have an explanatory force".[91] The use in this present study of
oral testimony serves to remind the historian that a profession is very much a group of people and not a collection of
criteria; such evidence helps to raise as many questions as it
might answer, but in saying this it is not the intention "to
exalt one kind of evidence over another, but to propose a continuous interplay between them, and a more extended use of
both."[92]

The use of oral evidence appears to excite considerable
anxiety among some historians, or perhaps the way such evidence is used is what excites them;[93] few have felt the need
to worry about the use of fiction in historical analysis.[94]
In part this is because few historians consciously make use of
fiction except in studies of reading, education or 'culture';
it is, perhaps, also because those works of fiction which do
creep into historical discussions tend to be those from what
we might describe as serious, classical, or 'haute' literature,
that is, 'the great masters' tradition of English literature.

Some social historians and social scientists have made
considerable use of works of fiction as sources for analysis
of historical events or periods; in this group we may include
the studies by Neff (1929); Phillips and Tomkinson (1927);
Cazamian (1903) and more recently, Basch (1974).[95] Each of
these studies used novels as a source for the social history
of a period or of a particular section of society, such as
women, or a specific occupation, such as governessing.[96]

One reason why historians seem less anxious about using
novels as source is the apparent interchangeability of the
historical event or personality and the fictional representation: Rockwell has argued succinctly that human beings appear
to prefer education through parables, and that fictional
characters often acquire the status of real people or the
status of commonsense substitutes for real people.[97] Examples
of this process may be seen by the ease that the name Shylock
has become synonymous for anyone suspected of sharp financial
practice and parsimony, or in the case of nursing, the ease
with which the old style of nursing has become associated with
Sairey Gamp, until she now appears to be as 'real' as Florence
Nightingale herself.[98]

Fiction not only introduces new elements into the public
mind and thus "modifies attitudes",[99] it can also so overlay
'reality' as to take its place. A study of fiction can therefore tell the historian much about contemporary attitudes and
values, inform a study of what Lucien Goldman has called the

"processes of structuration and destruction".[100] By using
novels which discuss contemporary nurses and nursing systems,
we can trace the way in which nurses and the new nursing order
were regarded by specific groups and classes during the period
of social and occupational change. While the data relating to
work practices may be in short measure in the novel, that absence can speak just as loud as its inclusion; it tells us,
for example, that many contemporaries feared less the changing
technical nature of nursing and more the substitution of
every-woman as nurse by a new trained professional. The novel,
then, can enhance our discussion of occupational imperialism:
while we should not rely solely on them, nor expect the novels
to be exact mirror images of reality, "it is true, and very
important to the social historian, that the spontaneous assumptions in the literature of any age, the behaviour of the
minor characters, the conventions against which irony and hu-
mour must be understood, reveal with great precision facts of
considerable interest about the structure of society."[101]

Each chapter of this study utilises a variety of source
material; the discussion of recruitment which makes up Chapter
2 relies, in particular, on original hospital records and oral
testimony; Chapter 3 concerns itself with the training and
socialisation of the nurse and draws upon data from nursing
textbooks, Parliamentary Reports and other printed sources. In
Chapter 4 the post-certification experiences of general nurses
are examined to illustrate the way in which this group of
nurses came to dominate the heterogeneous occupation, and
makes use of contemporary records and registers. Chapter 5 is
mainly concerned with whether the new nurses were 'better'
than the old, that is whether the new nurses were more skilled
in the care of and the treatment of illness than the nurses
they replaced; for much of that data we shall use contemporary
fiction as a counterweight to occupational polemic. Each chapter will, however, make use of material from a variety of
sources without giving primacy to any particular one. Before
we look in detail at nursing, however, it would be pertinent
to briefly outline the major changes in women's work which
have some bearing on the changes taking place in nursing in
the period 1881 - 1914.

NOTES

1. G. B. Shaw, The Doctor's Dilemma (Constable, London,
1913), Act 1.
2. The differences between types of hospitals and
definitions of hospitals are given in R. Pinker, English
Hospital Statistics 1861 - 1938 (Heinemann, London, 1966),
pp. 1-2. See also, Woodward, To Do The Sick No Harm, pp. 36-8;
Abel-Smith, Nursing Profession, p.3.
3. Evidence of Dr. Bedford Fenwick, Select Committee on
Registration of Nurses, 1905, vii, p.2.

4. H. C. Burdett, Hospitals and the State (Churchill, London, 1881), p.8.

5. Evidence of H. C. Burdett, Select Committee on Registration of Nurses, 1904, vi, p.142.

6. Davies, 'Where Next?', pp. 920-2. See also C. Davies (editor), Rewriting Nursing History (Croom Helm, London, 1980), pp. 11-14.

7. Abel-Smith, Nursing Profession, Chapters V - VII.

8. Woodward, To Do The Sick No Harm, p.51.

9. For example, L. Holcombe, Victorian Ladies at Work: Middle-class Working Women in England and Wales 1850 - 1914 (David and Charles, Newton Abbot, 1973), pp. 68-70.

10. Woodward, To Do The Sick No Harm, p.144.

11. Burdett, Directory, 1898; E. C. Vernet, 'Hospital Management', in (various authors), Science and Art of Nursing (Cassells, London, 1908), p. 129; R. White, Social Change and the Development of the Nursing Profession: A Study of the Poor Law Nursing Service 1848 - 1948 (Kimpton, London, 1978), pp. 85-6, pp. 228-9; F. B. Smith, The People's Health 1830 - 1910 (Croom Helm, London, 1979), pp. 270-71.

12. H. C. Burdett, Hints in Sickness: Where to Go and What to Do (Kegan Paul, Trench, London, 1883), pp. 121-6.

13. Abel-Smith, Nursing Profession, Appendix 1, pp. 253-59; Holcombe, Victorian Ladies at Work, Appendix pp. 204-5; A. L. Chapman and P. Knight, Wages and Salaries in the U.K. 1920 - 1938 (C.U.P., London, 1953), pp. 187-192.

14. Burdett, Registration of Nurses, 1905, p. 102; Abel-Smith, Nursing Profession, p. 255; G. Routh, Occupations and Pay in Great Britain 1906 - 60 (Cambridge University Press, London, 1965), p. 16.

15. H. M. Simpson, 'The Influence of Professional Nursing on the Development of the Modern Hospital' in F. N. L. Poynter (editor), The Evolution of Hospitals, (Pitman, London, 1964), p. 245; White, Social Change, pp. 213-16; Smith, People's Health, pp. 260-2.

16. Woodward, To Do The Sick No Harm, Chapter 10; Smith, People's Health, pp. 249-78, pp. 280-84; A. Hake, Suffering London (Scientific Press, London, 1892), pp. 109 et seq.

17. R. White, 'The Development of the Poor Law Nursing Service 1848 - 1948: A Discussion of the Historical Method and a Summary of some of the Findings', International Journal of Nursing Studies, 14, (1), 1977, p. 25, p. 29; White, Social Change, p. 214. See also, H. Balme, A Criticism of Nursing Education (O.U.P., Oxford, 1937), pp. 13 - 14; G. B. Carter, A New Deal for Nurses (Gollancz, London, 1939), p. 57, p. 148; R. Pomeranz, The Lady Apprentices: A Study of transition in nurse training (Occasional Papers in Social Administration 51, Bell, London, 1973), pp. 19-20; Baly, Nursing and Social Change, p. 164.

18. Holcombe, Victorian Ladies at Work pp. 72-5; Woodward, To Do The Sick No Harm, pp. 30-5; Smith, People's Health, pp.

260-2. See also, Sir E. Cook, Florence Nightingale (MacMillan, London, 1913); C. Woodham-Smith, Florence Nightingale (Constable, London, 1950).

19. Baly, Nursing and Social Change, pp. 140-1; Abel-Smith, Nursing Profession, pp. 99-113; C. Davies, 'The Regulation of Nursing Work: An Historical Comparison of Britain and the U.S.A.', Research in the Sociology of Health Care, Vol. 2, 1982, p. 129.

20. Kalisch and Kalisch, American Nursing, p. 1.

21. F. Nightingale, 'Training of Nurses and Nursing the Sick Poor' in R. Quain, Dictionary of Medicine (Longmans, Green, London, 1882), p. 237.

22. F. Nightingale, Notes on Nursing: What it is and What it is not (1860) (Morris reprint, London, 1946), np. See also, B. Ehrenreich and D. English, For Her Own Good: 150 Years of the Expert's Advice to Women (Doubleday, New York, 1979), Chapters Two and Five.

23. H. Martineau, 'Female Industry', Edinburgh Review, CIX, 1859, pp. 293-336; W. R. Grey, Why are Women Redundant? (London, 1869); B. L. Hutchings, Women in Modern Industry (Bell, London, 1915), p. 75, Chapter III; D. Haynes, 'A comparative Study of the Occupations of Men and Women', Women's Industrial News, XIX, New Series, 71, October 1915, pp. 365-414; W. Neff, Victorian Working Women: A Historical and Literary Study of Women in British Industries and Professions 1832-1850 (Allen and Unwin, London, 1966), pp. 11-14; Holcombe, Victorian Ladies at Work, pp. 10-12; P. Branca, Silent Sisterhood: Middle-Class Women in the Victorian Home (Croom Helm, London, 1975) (1977 edition), pp. 1-4; P. Branca, Women in Europe since 1750 (Croom Helm, London, 1978), Chapter 2; A Hammerton, Emigrant Gentlewomen: Genteel Poverty and Female Emigration 1830 - 1914 (Croom Helm, London, 1979), pp. 28 - 34.

24. E. Gamarnikow, 'Sexual Division of Labour: The case of nursing' in A. Kuhn and A. Wolpe (editors), Feminism and Materialism (Routledge, London, 1978), p. 102.

25. Dr. Bedford Fenwick was Honorary Surgeon at several London hospitals including The London Hospital for Women. Ethel Gordon Manson (Mrs. Bedford Fenwick) was trained as a nurse at the Manchester Royal Infirmary (1878), and appointed matron at Bart's (1881) aged 24. She founded the British Nurses Association and edited The Nursing Record. See W. Hector, Mrs. Bedford Fenwick (R.C.N., London, 1973); Abel-Smith, Nursing Profession, pp. 62-80.

26. Dr. Fenwick, Registration of Nurses, 1905, pp. 174-80.

27. Ibid., p. 111.

28. Dr. Fenwick, Registration of Nurses, 1904, pp. 3-4. See also, Nightingale, 'Training of Nurses', p. 232; Gamarnikow, 'Sexual Division of Labour', pp. 115-6.

29. Gamarnikow, 'Sexual Division of Labour', pp. 110-11.

30. C. Saleeby, Woman and Womanhood, (Heinemann, London,

1909), p. 17.

31. Branca, Women, pp. 51-2.

32. Nursing was little different in this respect from other white blouse work. For examples of such work see, Branca, Women, pp. 51-68; A. Davin, 'Telegraphists and Clerks', Bulletin of the Society for the Study of Labour History, 26, Spring 1973, pp. 7-9.

33. Davies, 'Regulation', pp. 121-3.

34. P. Stearns, Lives of Labour: Work in a Maturing Industrial Society (Croom Helm, London, 1975), pp. 46-7, pp. 59-61. (This list is by no means exhaustive).

35. M. Voysey, Nursing: Hints to Probationers on Practical Work (Scientific Press, London, 1901) (1905 edition), pp. 3-5. See also, L. Maule, 'Training Schools and Other Institutions' in Science and Art of Nursing, pp. 48-9.

36. A. Hughes, 'Nursing as a Vocation' in Science and Art of Nursing, p. 95.

37. Maule, 'Training Schools', p. 48. For a recent comment on the 'best' age to nurse see, Abel-Smith, Nursing Profession, p. 123.

38. Guy's Hospital Nursing Guide (Ash, London, 1904) pp. 5-6.

39. Ibid., p. 6.

40. Hughes, 'Nursing', p. 95.

41. Ibid., p. 95. It may also be that the older recruit would be less susceptible to discipline.

42. Ibid., p. 95.

43. Gamarnikow, 'Sexual Division of Labour', pp. 111-13.

44. M. Vivian, Lectures to Nurses in Training (Scientific Press, London, 1920), p. 9; Guy's Hospital, p. 7.

45. Maule, 'Training Schools', p. 58.

46. Vivian, Lectures, pp. 7-9.

47. Ibid., p. 10; Maule, 'Training Schools', p. 49.

48. Guy's Hospital, p. 7; Vivian, Lectures, pp. 7-9.

49. Vivian, Lectures, p. 7, gives the (qualified) exceptions.

50. Ibid., p. 8.

51. Ibid., pp. 7-8.

52. Burdett, Directory, 1898.

53. Voysey, Hints, p. 4.

54. "She should be well read in standard books. Elementary arithmetic is necessary in relation to the measuring of medicines and calculating doses. A knowledge of Latin (elementary) is not essential, but is of great assistance in understanding prescriptions and medical terms generally." Voysey, Hints, p. 4.

55. Burdett, Directory, 1898.

56. J. Gathorne-Hardy, The Public School Phenomenon, 597-1977 (Penguin, London, 1979), Chapters 10 - 13.

57. Davin, 'Telegraphists', p. 7.

58. Mrs. Bedford Fenwick, 'Nursing Echoes', British

Journal of Nursing, 29 September, 1906, pp. 251-2.

59. Voysey, Hints, pp. 3-5.

60. Evidence of Miss Hobbs, Select Committee on Registration of Nurses, 1904, vi, p. 72. See also, Evidence of Miss Kent, Select Committee on Registration of Nurses, 1905, vii, Appendix 4, p. 181.

61. Kent, Registration of Nurses, 1905, p. 181, Holcombe, Victorian Ladies at Work, p. 75; F. Nightingale, 'Letter to Probationer-Nurses in the 'Nightingale Fund' Training School at St. Thomas's Hospital' cited in Gamarnikow, 'Sexual Division of Labour', p. 117.

62. Gamarnikow, 'Sexual Division of Labour', pp. 119-20.

63. Ibid., pp. 112-14.

64. Abel-Smith, Nursing Profession, pp. 19-23; Holcombe, Victorian Ladies at Work, pp. 75-7.

65. Cited in W. Brockbank, The History of Nursing at the Manchester Royal Infirmary (M.U.P., Manchester, 1970), p. 63.

66. Mrs. O. Chant, 'Nursing Scrubbers', Nursing Record, 12 January, 1893, p. 29.

67. Lady Priestly, 'Nurses a la Mode', Nineteenth Century, January 1897, pp. 28-30.

68. Nightingale, Notes on Nursing, p. 11.

69. Brockbank, M.R.I., pp. 64-5.

70. 'The Truth about Infirmary Nursing', Nursing Mirror, 14 September, 1907, p. 361.

71. Late Matron, 'Necessary and Unnecessary Ward Work', The Hospital, 16 November 1901, pp. 98-9. (The author was probably Miss I.Stewart, ex-matron of Bart's).

72. Gamarnikow, 'Sexual Division of Labour', pp. 119 et seq.

73. Holcombe, Victorian Ladies at Work, p. 76; Abel-Smith, Nursing Profession, p. 24.

74. R. Nash (Editor), Florence Nightingale to Her Nurses (MacMillan, London, 1914), p. 14. See also, Miss Morris, 'Introductory Lecture', Nursing Times, 17 August 1907, p. 712 "He who rules over free men must himself be free".

75. Late Matron, 'Ward Work', p. 99.

76. M. Petersen, The Medical Profession in Mid-Victorian London (University of California Press, London, 1978); N. Parry and J. Parry, The Rise of the Medical Profession: A Study of Collective Social Mobility, (Croom Helm, London, 1976).

77. Parry and Parry, Medical Profession, Chapters 6 - 7.

78. See, for example, Sir A. Conan Doyle, The Stark Munro Letters. Being a Series of twelve letters written by J. S. M., MB., to his friend and former fellow student, Herbert Swanborough of Lowell, Mass., during the years 1881 - 84. (Longmans, Green, London, 1895).

79. 'Women as Nurses': A Doctor's Amazement', Bristol Evening Post, 2 August 1910, p. 3.

80. Holcombe, Victorian Ladies at Work, p. 77.

81. J. Donnison, Midwives and Medical Men. A History of

Inter-Professional Rivalries and Women's Rights (Heinemann, London, 1977).

82. White, Social Change, pp. 88-90; G. Trelawney, In a Cottage Hospital (Werner, Laurie, London, 1901); E. J. R. Landale, 'Nursing in a Workhouse Infirmary', Nursing Record, 6 January 1894, pp. 6-8.

83. Abel-Smith, Nursing Profession, pp.· 24-5.

84. Hake, Suffering London, p. 161; see also, A Sister, A Life in Hospital (Nisbet, London, nd.); Laurence, Nurse's Life, pp. 81-2.

85. See C. Davies (editor), 'Introduction' to M. Carpenter, 'Asylum Nursing before 1914: A Chapter in the History of Labour', in C. Davies (editor), Rewriting Nursing History (Croom Helm, London, 1980), p. 123.

86. For a discussion of the use of hospital archives and nursing history see, J. Foster and J. Sheppard, 'Archives and the History of Nursing', in Davies (Editor), Rewriting, pp. 200-14.

87. For example, A. Terton, Lights and Shadows in a Hospital (Methuen, London, 1902): F. F. Brook, Nursing in Many Fields (Johnson, London, 1977): F. Gilpin, Scenes from Hospital Life (Drane's, London, nd.); E. Haldane, British Nurse in Peace and War (Murray, London, 1923); G. M. Hardy, Yes, Matron (Beck, London, 1951); Laurence, Nurse's Life; E. Wilson, Gone with the Raj (Reeve, Norfolk, 1974); E. Davidson, 'A Career in Nursing a Century Ago', Nursing Mirror, 13 April, 1978, p. 58; R. Nettleton, 'A Nurse's Life in the 1900's', Nursing Times, 21 December 1972, p. 1615; M. Schofield, 'On A Summer's Day in 1879', Nursing Mirror, 4 June 1971, pp. 30-1; M. Stollard, 'Nursing on £12 a year', Yorkshire Post, 7 May 1962.

88. For example, R. Samuel, 'Local History and Oral History', History Workshop, 1, 1976; P. Thompson, The Voice of the Past: Oral History (O.U.P., London, 1978); P. Thompson, The Edwardians: The Remaking of British Society (Weidenfeld and Nicolson, London, 1975) (1977 edition).

89. B. Harrison, 'Oral History and Recent Political History', Oral History, 3, 1973, p. 46.

90. Thompson, The Edwardians; Thompson, Oral History, p. 47.

91. Samuel, 'Oral History', p. 204.

92. Ibid., p. 204.

93. See the criticisms voiced 'Editorial', Bulletin of the Society for the Study of Labour History, 27, Autumn, 1973, p. 3; also, Thompson, Oral History, p. 51.

94. Except, perhaps, P. Laslett, The World We Have Lost (Methuen, London, 1965) (1971 edition), pp. 90-1.

95. Neff, Victorian Working Women; M. Phillips and W. S. Tomkinson, English Women in Life and Letters: Women in the Professions (O.U.P., Oxford, 1927); L. Cazamain, The Social Novel in England 1830 - 1850; Dickens, Mrs. Gaskell, Kingsley

(Routledge and Kegan Paul, London, 1973) (originally 1903); F.
Basch, Relative Creatures: Victorian Women in Society and the
Novel 1837 - 67 (Allen Lane, London, 1974).
    96. See also, C. B. Needham and R. P. Utter, Pamela's
Daughters (Russell and Russell, New York, 1936) (1972 edi-
tion); B. Howe, A Galaxy of Governesses (Yerschoyle, London,
1959); D. Spearman, The Novel and Society (Routledge and
Kegan Paul, London, 1966); J. Rockwell, Fact in Fiction: The
Use of literature in the systematic study of society (Rout-
ledge and Kegan Paul, London, 1974); A. R. Cunningham, 'The
'New Woman' Fiction of the 1800's,'Victorian Studies, 17
December 1973, pp. 177-86; P. Stubbs, Women and Fiction:
Feminism and the Novel 1880 - 1920 (Harvester, Sussex, 1979);
P. Thomson, The Victorian Heroine: A Changing Ideal 1837 -
1873 (O.U.P., London, 1956); M. F. Brightfield, 'The Medical
Profession in Early Victorian England as depicted in the novels
of the period 1840 - 1870', Bulletin of the History of Medi-
cine, XXXV, 1961, pp. 238-56.
    97. Rockwell, Fact in Fiction, p. 27.
    98. Ibid., p. 3; also Phillips and Tomkinson, English
Women, p. 341, Basch, Relative Creatures, p. 145. A full dis-
cussion of this construct is given in K. Williams, 'From
Sarah Gamp to Florence Nightingale: A Critical Study of Hospital Nursing Systems from 1840 - 1897' in Davies (editor),
Rewriting, pp. 41-75.
    99. D. Spearman, 'The Social Influence of Fiction', New
Society, 6 July 1972, p. 6.
    100. Cited in Rockwell, Fact in Fiction, p. 4.
    101. Laslett, World We Have Lost, p. 90.

Appendix to Chapter 1

Women's "white blouse" work 1881 - 1914

If Mrs. Bedford Fenwick could have had her way entirely concerning recruitment to general nursing at the turn of the century, entry would have been restricted to those women who
could afford to pay for their training, in particular to the
"daughters of the higher social classes".[1] She wanted the new
generation of nurses to be drawn from "a class of women who
had been trusted for so many years that the failures would be
the exceptions".[2] These failures were not only those who were
unable to complete the technical part of their training but
also those who were morally unfit to practice, in particular
once they had left the enclosed and supportive world of the
general hospital.

Even the most ardent supporter of this line was forced
to admit that it could only result in a chronic shortage of
nurses, in-training and trained, since there were just not
enough such paragons willing to enter the "calling".[3] Consequently a more pragmatic recruitment policy, in which almost
anyone could begin training, ought to be counteracted by a
rigid training and examination system which, it was hoped,
would culminate in the recognition of the right to practice by
State Registration.

One of the practical reasons, although one not openly
admitted to, for allowing a more open entry to training was
that after the 1880's nursing found itself in the unenviable
and somewhat contradictory position of having to compete for
its recruits with other expanding and developing areas of
women's work. We need to briefly look at certain areas of that
expanding work opportunity market, if only because nursing may
have been only one of many similar areas of work open to women
in the period and that nursing, far from being a 'vocation' or
even a first-choice occupation, was one step in a series of
occupations undertaken by the sort of women we find as recruits
to nursing.[4]

Demographic change

Between 1861 and 1881 the total population of England and Wales

38

increased by approximately 29.44%, from 20,066,244 to
25,974,439 persons: between 1881 and 1911 the increase was
38.87%, to a total of 36,070,492 persons. Of these totals, females increased by 29.59% and 39.67% respectively, and males
by 29.29% and 38.02% respectively.[5] This general imbalance between the sexes, which first alarmed the Victorian middle-
classes in 1851,[6] is more clearly seen by comparing the ratio
of females per 1,000 males, and by extending that comparison
to include the ratios at specific age groups: that data is
summarised in Tables 1.4 - 1.6. While demographically all
groups are important, for this present study it is those
ratios in what we might refer to as the economically- and
maritally-significant age groups which will be discussed.

For the age groups 20-24; 25-29; and 30-34 years, that
is those most closely linked with the highest chances of marriage and the most economically productive years in terms of
work opportunities, females exceeded males in the census years
1881 - 1911 as follows

Age Group	1881	1891	1901	1911
20-24	1093	1122	1119	1113
25-29	1083	1115	1126	1115
30-34		1073	1100	1091

Source: Table 1.5, below

As these data suggest, the proportion of women who were
both single and aged 20-34 years rose between 1881 and 1901,
and rose at a higher rate than did men who were single and
aged 25-34 years. The general conclusion which such data present is that as the century drew to a close and well into the
first decade of the twentieth-century an increasing number of
women remained single in the age groups most usually associated with first-time marriage.[7] For many of these women, who
may or may not have been 'surplus' or 'redundant' to the needs
of men and marriage,[8] it was an economic necessity that they
work and chose work which could offer them long-term financial
support, if not security.

Employment changes
Not all of the women we have noted above were employed in the
period 1881 - 1914, since we can note a contemporaneous increase in the numbers of women who stayed at home;[9] however,
the data concerning female participation in the workforce
show a remarkably consistent proportion of occupied and unoccupied women in the general population between 1881 - 1911;
viz.

Table 1.4: Population, 1801 – 1921, England and Wales

Date of Enumeration	Population			Increase of Population since the Preceding Census			Decennial Increase per cent of population			No. of Females to 1000 Males
	Persons	Males	Females	Persons	Males	Females	Persons	Males	Females	
1801	8892536	4254735	4677801	-	-	-	-	-	-	1057
1811	10164256	4873605	5290651	1271720	618870	652850	14.00	14.24	13.78	1054
1821	12000236	5850319	6149917	1835980	976714	859266	18.06	20.03	16.23	1036
1831	13896797	6771196	7125601	1896561	920877	975684	15.80	15.73	15.86	1040
1841	15914148	7777586	8136562	2017351	10C6390	1010961	14.27	14.39	14.15	1046
1851	17927609	8781225	9146384	2013661	1003639	1009822	12.65	12.68	12.62	1042
1861	20066224	9776259	10239965	2138615	995034	1143881	11.90	11.30	12.47	1053
1871	22712266	11058934	11653332	2646042	1282675	1363367	13.21	13.74	13.27	1054
1881	25974439	12639902	13334537	3262173	1580968	1681205	14.36	14.29	14.42	1055
1891	29002525	14052901	14949624	3028086	1412999	1615087	11.65	11.17	12.11	1064
1901	32527843	15728613	16799230	3525318	1675712	1849606	12.17	11.94	12.39	1068
1911	36070492	17445608	18624884	3542649	1716995	1825654	10.89	10.91	10.86	1068
1921	37886699	18075239	19811460	1816207	629631	1186576	4.93	3.53	6.24	1096

Source: Table 1 Population, 1801 – 1921, England and Wales. : General Report, 1921 Census of Population, Part II – Population : 1, General, p. 12.

Table 1.5: Ratios of Females to 1000 males, England and Wales 1881 - 1911 at specific age groups

Ages	1881	1891	1901	1911
All Ages	1055	1064	1068	1068
0 - 4	1033	1010	1003	991
5 - 9	1007	1005	1005	1001
10 - 14	997	1001	1000	1003
15 - 19	1008	1014	1019	1016
20 - 24	1093	1122	1119	1113
25 - 29	1083	1115	1126	1115
30 - 34		1073	1100	1091
35 - 39	1074	1059	1074	1072
40 - 44		1075	1062	1077
45 - 49	1103	1082	1070	1079
50 - 54		1111	1089	1086
55 - 59	1123	1139	1116	1103
60 - 64		1166	1170	1138
65 - 69	1186	1203	1230	1205
70 - 74		1256	1283	1337
75 - 79	1275	1293	1339	1431
80 - 84		1416	1470	1556
85+	1602	1696	1699	1817

Sources: Table 14, Census 1881, Gen. Report, p. 89; Table XXX, Gen. Report, Census 1921, p. 61.

Table 1.6: Marital Conditions: Proportions of Females in Selected Age Groups, England and Wales, 1881 - 1911

Age	Status	1881	1891	1901	1911
15 and up	Single	367	387	395	390
	Married	517	499	497	506
	Widowed	116	114	108	104
15 - 19	Single	975	981	985	988
	Married	25	19	15	12
	Widowed	0	0	0	0
20 - 24	Single	665	701	726	757
	Married	331	296	272	242
	Widowed	4	3	2	1
25 - 34	Single	293	326	340	355
	Married	681	653	643	632
	Widowed	26	21	17	13
35 - 44	Single	153	164	185	196
	Married	765	761	751	753
	Widowed	82	75	64	51

Source: Table XLI, Census 1921, General Report p. 83.

41

25.53% occupied females per total female population 1881
25.54% .... do 1891
24.72% .... do 1901
25.60% .... do .... 1911[10]

Within these fairly constant proportions of occupied women to total population there are, however, hidden but important changes in the distribution of women in work, the major components of which are summarised in Tables 1.7 - 1.10, and further detailed in Table 1.11.

In general terms, there was a steady trend away from extractive occupations, including agriculture, fishing and mining (2.17 - 0.95%); an overall decline in the building-manufacturing trades (39.91 - 37.43%); and a significant expansion in the tertiary, service sector (57.92 - 61.62%), at a time when the number of occupied women remained fairly constant.[11]

Within the tertiary area, however, expansion was most remarkable in those occupations categorised by Hogg as Public Utilities; Commerce; Public Administration and to a lesser extent, Professional Services.[12] These areas of work are those which have been characterised as "white-blouse", and the expansion in that sector has been described by one historian of women's work as a "revolution", an epithet which adequately expresses contemporary impressions of such changes in opportunities for women to work.[13]

Since nursing falls into this sector and some, if not all, of its recruits might have considered such other areas of work for themselves or indeed have actually been drawn away from other such work, it would be pertinent to look at the major changes taking place in this sector of women's work in the period 1881 - 1914. We can therefore look at domestic service because many nurses were said to come from that group or from the 'class'; at clerical and commercial work because of its similarities of notions of gentility; and at elementary school teaching, because it also involved a training system, offered nursing a model for professionalisation through state regulation and was almost entirely a 'female' area of work. We shall be primarily concerned in this section with those features such as recruitment and conditions of service which have a direct bearing on our discussion of nursing.

Domestic Service

There is little doubt that one of the most singular features of the Victorian-Edwardian economy was that its greatest industry was not an 'industrial' one. In terms of numbers employed, it was the entirely non-industrial sector - domestic service - which led the field.[14]

Table 1.7: Percent females of total occupied population in
grouped sectors, England and Wales 1881 - 1911

Grouped Sectors	1881	1891	1901	1911
Agri-Fishing, Mining (1,2)	0.66	0.47	0.32	0.28
Building-Manufacture (3,4)	12.14	12.11	11.18	11.00
Services (5 - 9)	17.62	17.61	17.52	18.12
% of total occupied	30.42	30.19	29.02	29.40
% occupied of total population	13.10	13.17	12.77	13.22

Source: M. Ebery and B. Preston, Domestic Service in Late Victorian and Edwardian England 1871 - 1914 (University
of Reading, Reading, 1976), p. 17.

Table 1.8: Percent females of occupied females in 9 selected
sectors, England and Wales, 1881 - 1911

Sector	1881	1891	1901	1911
Agri-Fishing	1.91	1.36	0.93	0.81
Mining	0.26	0.20	0.17	0.14
Building	0.08	0.07	0.02	0.01
Manufacture	39.83	40.06	38.54	37.42
Transport	0.26	0.26	0.23	0.34
Dealing	6.12	7.81	8.75	12.33
Industrial Services	0.27	0.54	1.39	2.58
Public - Professional Services	5.85	6.95	8.04	8.63
Domestic Service	45.42	52.75	41.93	37.74
% of Total Occupied	100	100	100	100

Source: Ebery and Preston, Domestic Service, p. 19.

Table 1.9: Percent females of total occupied population in 9
selected sectors, England and Wales, 1881 - 1911

Sector	1881	1891	1901	1911
Agri-Fishing	0.58	0.41	0.27	0.24
Mining	0.08	0.06	0.05	0.04
Building	0.02	0.02	0.00	0.00
Manufacture	12.12	12.09	11.18	11.00
Transport	0.08	0.08	0.07	0.09
Dealing	1.86	2.33	2.54	3.63
Industrial Service	0.08	0.16	0.14	0.76
Public Professional Service	1.78	2.10	2.33	2.54
Domestic Service	13.82	12.90	12.17	11.10
% of Total Occupied	30.42	30.15	28.75	29.40

Source: Ebery and Preston, Domestic Service, p. 19.

Table 1.10: Female Participation in the Labour Force, England
and Wales 1881 - 1911, aged 15 years and over

	Occupational Order	1881	1891	1901	1911
1	General or Local Government	7314	14894	26367	44786
2	Defence	-	-	-	-
3	Professional + Sub Services	182037	236162	290174	245162
4	Domestic Offices + Services	1419042	1605914	1622619	1686616
5	Commercial Occups.	8339	20379	58592	124710
6	Conveyance of Men etc.	9925	12065	15618	25679
7	Agriculture	62089	49440	56315	92358
8	Fishing	276	313	163	98
9	Mines and Quarries	4144	2913	2286	2635
10	Metals, Machines etc.	34758	42466	59243	91531
11	Precious Metals etc.	9099	10588	14882	22301
12	Building and Construction	1827	2363	2338	4670
13	Wood, Furniture etc.	17638	18924	23463	29142
14	Brick, Cement etc.	22381	26481	30837	36410
15	Chemicals etc.	7289	13323	24797	38216
16	Skins, leathers etc.	14797	17845	23507	28412
17	Paper, Prints etc.	38891	58084	83254	114341
18	Textile Fabrics	544913	575651	601448	681679
19	Dress	587075	652620	680854	725396
20	Food, Tobacco etc.	158120	253185	292547	466872
21	Gas, Water etc.	179	157	113	99
22	Other General etc.	58166	64701	58470	83170
23	Unoccupied	5402117	6165795	7548391	8456815
	Total Occupied	3188299	3679368	3967887	4644283
	% occupied females over 15 years	37.1	37.4	34.5	35.4

Source: Table 26, Census 1911, pp. 540-51.

Table 1.11: Percentage Increase or Decrease of Female Workers in Great Britain, 1891 - 1911, by Industry, and Females as a percent of all workers, 1891 - 1911, by Industry

Industry	% Increase or Decrease 1891 - 1911	% Females of All Workers	
		1891	1911
Exceptional Expansion			
Public Utilities	644.44	0.02	0.08
Commerce	550.61	5.25	17.47
Public Administration	195.32	10.36	15.51
Chemicals, Oils etc.	166.74	19.72	25.25
Metals	107.21	4.85	6.30
Transport and Communications	93.24	1.76	2.36
Paper	91.23	30.21	37.14
Distribution	58.50	29.99	29.99
Skins and Leather	49.78	20.15	26.87
Professional Services	45.12	46.80	48.10
Food, Drink, Tobacco etc.	35.80	24.17	29.25
Bricks, Cement, Glass etc.	27.51	20.66	21.56
Exceptional Decline			
Mining	13.08	0.74	0.51
Personal Service	8.51	87.08	81.97
Clothing	3.81	65.21	68.30
Textiles	3.52	59.40	59.44
Agriculture and Fishing	-14.03	9.11	7.83
Miscell. Manufacture	-56.02	2.83	2.24
Construction	-72.73	0.30	0.06
Stable			
Wood	18.66	10.98	10.37
National Defence	-	-	-
Total All Workers	18.89	31.31	29.56

Source: S. Hogg, 'The Employment of Women in Great Britain, 1891 - 1921' (Unpublished D. Phil., University of Oxford, 1964), Table 30, p. 326a.

- thus a recent study of domestic service introduced the topic
to the reader. In total, the number of women employed as
domestic servants in some capacity at each census date between
1881 and 1911 never fell below 38% of all occupied women, even
though the percentage so employed had actually fallen from 45%
in 1881 to 38% in 1911 (approximately).

The decline in the total numbers of females occupied as
domestic servants was matched by a fall in the proportion of
female to male servants, which became more marked after 1901
and was almost entirely due to a decline in "private residence
employment" which added fuel to the general contemporary concern with the servant shortage.[16] According to the Report of
The War Cabinet Committee on Women in Industry (1919) women
who might have entered service were entering other types of
tertiary sector work, especially clerical work[17]; but the decline in the number of women working as indoor domestic servants was, that Report concluded, a result of an inter-occupa-
tional redistribution, whereby women chose non-residential
service in the "accommodation-refreshment" areas such as ho-
tels and guesthouses, and work in the public and private institutions, such as hospitals and offices.[18] Women continued
to work as domestic servants but preferred to work outside of
the homes of individual members of the servant-keeping classes.

Conditions of service among domestic servants varied
enormously not only between situations but between indoor,
resident posts and living-out positions. They depended upon
the employer's financial position ("the minimum wage needed to
keep a general maid was about £100 a year")[19]; space available
in the employer's home; whether other servants were kept; the
age and experience of the servant; the length of stay in the
post and the grade of employment.[20]

There was no single method of finding a servant or of a
servant finding a position.[21] The first post was frequently
found by the girl's parents, might indeed be in the home of a
sort of relative, but was usually in the home of a tradesman
or professional man in a nearby town.[22] This first post rarely
lasted more than two years and if the conditions experienced
by the girl were felt, to be unusually harsh or unfair, this
first job might only last a few weeks or so.[23]

The second and subsequent positions were obtained either
through word-of-mouth contacts, between employers and employees,
and between servants themselves, or through newspaper advertisements, or to some extent, through employment agencies, such
as the Metropolitan Association for Befriending Young Servants.
[24] These subsequent moves were generally made to get 'better'
situations where conditions of work, such as wages, free time,
or amount of work were improved. There were also attempts to
move up the servant hierarchy by moving between posts, and even
where the "objective conditions" did not improve following the
move, the change itself was seen by many servants as being
worthwhile and even an expression of the independence of the

servant.[25]

Data concerning wages paid to servants in England and Wales are poor and highly selective, and are only significant if compared to other areas of women's work when such variables as the cost of board and loding, position in the servant hierarchy, and the informal and complex relationships between employee and employer (which included tipping, hand-me-downs and 'poundage') are taken into account.[26] Table 1.12 summarises what remains an under-researched aspect of women's work, the actual wages received by servants in cash and in kind at the end of the nineteenth-century.

Domestic service employed well over one-third of all occupied women as enumerated at each census date, 1881 - 1911, and undoubtedly provided a temporary area of employment (which would be absent from census data) for many more women. While some married women remained as servants, (for example, 2% of all servants in 1851 were married),[27] the vast majority of servants, particularly indoor servants, were single women. Most servants did eventually marry, even if the age at which they did so was delayed compared to the national mean; it has therefore been argued that

> young women found servanthood a useful and respectable occupation before marriage and it enabled them to save money which could be used ... when they married ... English servants, like the French, often deliberately entered service with the intention of marrying well. Their chief contacts ... were with other servants, soldiers and sailors or the shopkeepers and artisans who supplied their employers' households.[28]

The popularity of the occupation cannot be explained by reference to the conditions of service - since pay could be very low and hours of work very long - but to the role this type of work played in the transition from one culture to another, rural to urban or later urban lower-working-class to urban-upper-working- and perhaps even lower-middle-calss.[29] Domestic service also held out the possibility of easing the transition from one home, the parental one, to another, the marriage home, and the possibility for discovering other areas of work. The emphasis in servanthood on the personal relationships between employer and employee was important to a young girl leaving home for the first time. She might reject domestic service when she discovered that she could get such relationships in other areas of work which appeared to have less of the disadvantages of service, or to set up her own home and family.[30] It is no wonder, then, that contemporaries emphasised the links between domestic service and nursing, both in the work performed by each and the type of women found in each. Both occupations stressed "human contacts" as integral parts

Table 1.12: Wages of female domestic servants at various ages, England and Wales (excluding London) Wage-index for 1899 (after Collett 1899)

Type of Servant

Age of Servant	General Servant	Cook	Housemaid	Parlour-Maid	Nurse a.	Lady's Maid	Kitchen Maid	Laundry Maid	House-keeper
15	100.0	-	123.1	-	98.5	-	90.8	-	-
16	118.5	-	147.7	-	146.2	-	133.9	-	-
17	144.6	130.8	170.8	200.0	164.6	-	161.5	-	-
18	170.8	176.9	196.9	215.4	170.8	161.5	189.2	-	-
19	181.5	210.8	198.5	269.2	169.2	-	183.1	-	-
20	184.6	247.7	223.1	253.9	224.6	292.3	230.8	246.2	-
21-24	224.6	269.2	249.2	280.0	253.9	300.0	255.4	260.0	-
25-29	244.6	310.8	284.6	316.9	309.2	380.0	323.1	363.1	-
30-34	263.1	338.5	310.8	323.1	338.5	380.0	-	369.2	580.0
35-39	238.5	375.4	315.4	353.8	346.2	387.6	-	400.0	-
40	227.7	376.9	313.9	316.9	398.5	384.6	-	353.9	803.1
Total Servants	276	648	813	219	199	86	115	23	9

Source: Ebery and Preston, Domestic Service, p. 97, citing C. Collett, Money Wages of Indoor Domestic Servants, Parliamentary Papers, 1899, XCll, pp. 25-26.

a. Not sick nurses

of the work experience, and both occupations set out to recruit first-time workers although perhaps for different reasons.

Clerical and Commercial Work

In 1861 there were approximately 279 female clerks and 91,733
male clerks; by 1881 the numbers had increased to 6,420 females and 229,705 males, representing an increase of over
2,000% for females and 150% for males. Such a percentage increase in females employed as clerks appears dramatic, but the
true extent of the feminisation of clerical work does not show
as far as census data are concerned until 1911 when 124,843
women were recorded as being employed as clerks in England and
Wales.[31]

In one major sense the expansion of women's clerical work
- the "revolution in clerical ... work"[32] - was delayed until
the invention and widespread use of technological innovations,
such as shorthand ('invented' circa 1888) and the typewriter
(1868).[33] The growth of commercial enterprises, banking, in-
surance, communications, the expansion of local and national
government and bureaucracy, and the increasing mechanisation
of office work which in turn required a lower standard of
general education, led to considerable specialisation and
division of labour based on gender within the business and
administrative worlds.[34] However, as Anderson cautions, this
development did not necessarily mean the displacement of male
by female workers, particularly in the commercial sector where
women "fulfilled an essentially different work function within
the office than men".[35]

With the increased demand for clerical and commercial
labour, the demise of what had been essentially an apprenticeship structure within male clerical work,[36] and the general
improvement in the basic level of education throughout society,
women could be and were drawn into this sector.[37] Between 1861
and 1911 the number of male clerks had increased by a factor
of 5; the number of female clerks by a factor of 400.[38] As we
have noted, however, it was not simply a case of displacement,
female clerical work being largely confined to the new commercial offices and businesses rather than being distributed
throughout the more traditional areas such as banking, insur-
ance, and the railway offices.[39]

Various explanations were offered for this development,
including the idea that women were more suited to using the
typewriter because of the size and shape of their fingers;[40]
the temperamental ability of women to accept routine and repe-
titious work,[41] and the association between middle-class women
who had first entered some of the areas of this work and the
status of female clerks in general.[42]

For many women clerical and commercial work offered important physical and social advantages over both manual and
domestic work; it was relatively easy and light work and

offered (even if it did not always supply) the possibility of acquiring middle-class culture, values and respectability.[43] The expansion of female clerical and commercial work was as much due to a change in attitudes to work on the part of the middle-classes, many of whom were the employers of this new group of workers and the daughters of whom sometimes took up the work in the early period.[44] The notions of gentility, good deportment and good speech were seen by employers as important qualifications for the work, and in turn helped to create and reinforce the status of the work as 'genteel'. The conditions under which many clerks lived, in 'homes' run by the employers or even in the employer's family in the early years and in the smaller establishments, tended to reinforce paternalistic attitudes to women at work in the clerical and commercial offices, which encouraged not only the girls to turn to them for employment but made the reluctance of the parents less tenable.[45]

However, the reverse was more usually the case; many typists and general clerks were ill-educated girls "who fly to typewriting and shorthand in preference to domestic service or a place behind the counter".[46] Their conditions of work were harder and more routine, their pay lower and their hours often longer than other areas of women's work.[47] These women formed a crucial element of the contemporary sweated trades,[48] but they still flocked to them drawn by the "gentility of the typists calling" which seemed to offer them a new world and appeared to form a reward in itself.[49]

While the growth in the scale of commerce and business, in all its forms, undoubtedly encouraged the feminisation of clerical and commercial work, perhaps the more important reasons for this expansion were the undoubted cheapness of female labour and, following the experiences of the unrest amongst male clerks and telegraphists at the end of the century, the apparent "docility" of white-blouse workers.[50]

One important feature of contemporary clerical and commercial work which has a bearing on our discussion of nursing in the same period is the operation of a marriage bar throughout most of this sector of women's work. This to some degree reflected contemporary attitudes to married women's work by the middle-classes,[51] but it also reflected the concern of employers, private company or State, to keep costs as low as possible in the operation of this aspect of their activities.

Within the private commercial and business sector the marriage bar, which required women to leave work when they chose to marry, was an informal but extensive practice. Many employers insisted that female employees leave on marriage, and this in turn reinforced their contention that such workers should be paid less and have lower status within the company and the sector than male workers. It was, they argued, easier to replace a relatively inexperienced and untrained junior than to replace a long-serving and skilled senior worker; women were therefore not trained beyond the basic skills needed for their functions within the lower echelons of the organisation and there were few opportunities for such women to progress up the hierarchy.[52]

The financial considerations went deeper than the cost of replacing women workers at the higher grades; employers argued that by imposing a marriage bar they would prevent many women from becoming eligible for a retirement pension, which, in view of the numbers of women employed as clerks (even if only some continued to work after marriage if they had the choice), could be a considerable cost factor over the whole sector.[53]

In the Post Office and in other areas of Government employment, the marriage bar was a formal requirement of contract, introduced by the Post Office circa 1875, other areas following suit from the 1890's onwards.[54] Unlike the private sector, however, there was a provision in the State sector for payment of a gratuity on 'retirement' due to marriage, as long as the woman had served for a minimum of six years.[55] Despite this apparent cost, the marriage bar in public service operated as it did in the private sector, to reduce long-term costs, although some contemporaries saw in the gratuity system a positive reason for women to enter the ranks of the civil service, providing such women with "a nice little dowry".[56]

Whatever the rationale for its operation or for the mixed reactions to it, the marriage bar effectively ensured that this sector of female employment was populated by young, single women, (occasionally by widows, rarely by married women) and increasingly by unmarried older women who had chosen to make a career out of the work. Or rather, the operation of the marriage bar together with the demographic changes noted earlier made clerical and commercial work one important area of employment where older unmarried women might find a niche for themselves which provided not only some degree of job-security and gentility but also the possibility of upward occupational mobility to supervisory levels. It also offered these 'spinsters', especially after the male-led agitation of the turn of the century,[57] the very real possibility of a reasonable pension on retirement and hence some measure of security in their old age.

Elementary School Teaching

Teaching was a heterogenous occupation, just as nursing, it encompassed different skills and knowledge and was provided at different levels, from the nursery governess to the university lecturer. In this study it is the elementary schoolteacher with whom we shall be concerned, in part because she (and he) formed the numerically significant section of the occupation, at least after the 1870 Education Act.[58]

Estimates of the numbers of elementary schoolteachers give figures of 23,656 in 1875, and 165,901 in 1914; of these women formed 54.3% and 74.5% of all elementary schoolteachers respectively. In 1875, therefore, there were approximately 12,845 women elementary schoolteachers and 123,596 in 1914, an over-all increase of 862.2%, and three times the rate of increase among male elementary schoolteachers.[59]

Most elementary schoolteachers received their training through an apprenticeship system, the pupil-teacher scheme whereby the candidate spent five years working under a quali-fied teacher after leaving school aged 13 years.[60] It was in-tended that this five-year apprenticeship would be followed by a formal and concentrated training at a teacher-training col-lege for two years; in practice the number of places available at such colleges was totally inadequate to meet the demands for admission.[61] Those pupil teachers who had served their time but could not find a college place became 'uncertificated teachers', with the possibility of being external candidates for certification.[62] In 1875 57% of all female elementary schoolteachers were trained and certificated, but by 1914 this had fallen to 32%.[63]

There existed a third tier of elementary schoolteacher, in addition to the certificated and uncertificated, known as "Article 68" or Supplementary teachers; these were women who

had to be over 18, to have been vaccinated, and to be able to satisfy the inspectors on their classroom proficiency. Many were married to headmasters, most were employed with the youngest children who were far more numerous in the school then.[64]

In 1900 there were about 20,000 Supplementary teachers, making up 22.5% of all female elementary schoolteachers;[65] as Table 1.13 shows, this number fell as the century progressed, although by 1910 they still formed 13% of all female, and 10% of the total number of elementary schoolteachers. By 1914 the proportions were 11% and 8% respectively.[66]

A new scheme had been introduced in 1907 in order to in-crease the recruitment to this level of education. The bursary system, provided for under the Education Act (1902) enabled pupils to remain at school and complete their own education until 17 or 18 when they could enter a training college.[67] It would appear, however, that the small amounts paid as bursa-ries; the delay bursars experienced before earning real wages and the increasingly wider career choices available to such well-educated women acted against the interests of the system and helped to create a short-fall in the numbers of intending teachers particularly in the years 1909 - 1913.[68]

The distinctions between the various grades of teachers were evident not only in their training and the type of chil-dren they taught, but in the salaries received. Wages varied according to grade and also by geographical area and the finan-cial restraints felt by local schoolmanagers; wages also varied by gender.[69] In a contemporary guide to women's work,[70]

Table 1.13: Numbers of Teachers of Various Grades in Public Elementary Schools 1910 - 1914, England and Wales

Date	Certificated		Uncertificated		Supplementary		Totals		Total
	Men	Women	Men	Women	Men	Women	Men	Women	
1909-10	32805	64591	6005	39550	-	15732	38810	119873	158683
1910-11	34255	67125	6137	39510	-	14408	40392	121043	161435
1911-12	34904	68609	5431	38632	-	13863	40735	121104	161839
1912-13	35990	70035	5303	37590	-	13477	41293	121102	162395
1913-14	37226	71930	4655	36752	-	13367	41881	122049	163930

Source: A. Oram, 'The Employment of Women Teachers 1910 - 1938' (Unpublished Paper, University of Bristol, 1978), citing Board of Education, Annual Reports and Statistics of Public Education for respective years.

Lady Dilke gave the following examples of wages paid to tea-chers:

Average Salaries of Certificated Mistresses, not
Principals (1893)

Denominations	Average Salary, including all professional sources of income £.s.d.	Numbers in Sample	Numbers Provided with House	
Nat. Soc. or C. of E. Schools	48 : 15 : 1	2520	150	
Wesleyan Schools	49 : 6 : 0	220	1	
R. C. Schools	50 : 4 : 2	477	7	
Brit. Undenomi-national and Others	54 : 10 : 3	533	5	
Board Schools	78 : 19 : 8	7591	31	
Total	69 : 6 : 7	11341	194	71

(A more recent description of teachers' wages is provided by the historian of teaching, Asher Tropp,[72] and these appear in Table 1.14).

A brief look at elementary school teaching has two other elements which offer important comparisons in our study of general nursing; they are the recruitment of trainee teachers and the demands within the occupation for professional status and state regulation.

According to a recent historian of women teachers,[73] the majority of female elementary schoolteachers came as recruits from the ranks of the working-classes, and many of those who entered this field might previously have gone into service or even factory work. Such recruits "eagerly took advantage of this expanding field of employment to better their economic position and as they considered it, to rise in the social scale".[74] The absence of a need for certification in order to practice and the number of unqualified supplementary teachers certainly lends weight to the view that access to the lower grades of teaching was more open to working-class women and that "elementary schools recruited their teachers almost en-tirely from their own ranks", that is their own schoolchildren through the pupil teacher system.[75]

Partington has argued recently (1976) that teaching was popular among women because it was "highly congruent with feminine roles and work styles".[76] A sample of elementary

Table 1.14: Average Annual Salary of Certificated Teachers (£'s)

Year	Male	Female
1855	90	61
1860	94	62
1865	87	55
1870	93½	57
1875	109	65
1880	121	73
1885	121	74
1890	120	76

Year	Male Average	Female Average	Male Head	Male Assistant	Female Head	Female Assistant
1895	122½	80	137	97	86	72½
1900	125½	84½	144	102½	94	76½
1905	130	88	145	110	100	82
1910	145	100	172	125½	121½	91½
1914	147	103	177	129	126	96
1918	180	128	195	170	155	120

Source: A. Tropp, The School Teachers (Heinemann, London, 1957), Appendix B, Table 1, p. 273.

schoolteachers working between 1900 and 1925 would seem to
bear out this stereotypical generalisation:[77] Miss H. said she
"chose to be a teacher first of all (because) I was so devoted
to children - I thought I was going to do something with
little children". Another said that she had played at being a
teacher when a child and that had helped to determine her in
her choice of career; for some women, apparently, there was
little choice between teaching and nursing - "the only thing
in those days you were either a teacher or a nurse" - and many
appear to have just "drifted" into the teaching profession.[78]
   Recruitment of elementary schoolteaching relied heavily
on parental pressure and the recommendation of the pupil's
head teacher. Widdowson's study has highlighted the concern,
by the mothers of women elementary schoolteachers especially,
for some girls to make good.[79] The parents of women interviewed in that study were essentially lower-middle-class, but
perhaps because of their own achievements - "she felt that
they had got somewhere" - their daughters were encouraged to
go into teaching either to obtain a training useful in widow-
hood or even during married life; or to get a pension, or to
achieve personal security through making a better marriage.[80]
   An aspect of the attraction of elementary schoolteaching
which played an important part in convincing many parents that
it was suitable work for their daughters was the increasing
social status and prestige being accorded to teachers in general and certificated teachers in particular. This development
was crystalised by the 1902 Act and the registration scheme it
embodied, a move welcomed by those in nursing who were looking
for similar developments.[81]
   The teachers' registration movement was important because
it served to unite a disparate occupation - elementary, specialist and secondary schoolteachers - behind a "great co-operative effort" to better their status and conditions of service.[82] The State scheme of registration, however, served only
to reinforce the distinctions between grades of teachers and
as a "miserable fiasco" it was abandoned in 1907.[83] A second
attempt to set up a register was made in 1912, which lasted
until 1949, but unlike those in nursing and medicine, the teachers' scheme never became effective guides to 'professional'
status or competence.[84]
   Elementary schoolteaching, and also secondary schoolteaching after the 1902 Education Act, was a popular career
choice for an increasing number of women from both the working-classes and from the ranks of the lower-middle-classes,
between 1880 and 1914. It has been argued that teaching provided a "psychologically satisfying outlet for the unmarried",
[85] and the operation of a marriage bar by most education
authorities tended to make it attractive to the increasing
number of older single women noted earlier.[86] Whether teaching
was a 'natural sphere' for women or not, (and even the femi-
nists themselves held many opinions on this point),[87] it was

undoubtedly a socially-approved area of work for women in the period. As such it, like domestic service, clerical and commercial work and even shopwork,[88] became an important and expanding area of possible job-choice for contemporary women. Nursing, then, may be seen as yet another such choice and not necessarily an occupation chosen because of a vocation or calling to the work. The next Chapter will therefore look in some detail at how nursing set about recruiting its trainees in the period 1881 - 1914.

NOTES

1. Abel-Smith, Nursing Profession, p. 57.
2. Evidence of Mrs. Bedford Fenwick, Select Committee on Registration of Nurses, 1905, vii, p. 33; Abel-Smith, Nursing Profession, pp. 62-3.
3. Abel-Smith, Nursing Profession, pp. 62-3.
4. L. Broom and J. H. S. Smith, 'Bridging Occupations', British Journal of Sociology, XLV, (4), December, 1963, pp. 321-34; Stearns, Lives of Labour, pp. 59-61.
5. General Report, Census of Population 1921, Table 1 Population 1801 - 1921, England and Wales, p. 12. See Table 1.4, above.
6. Martineau, 'Female Industry', pp. 293-336.
7. General Report, Census of Population 1921, p. 82. See also, J. A. Banks, Prosperity and Parenthood: A Study of Family Planning among the Victorian Middle Classes (Schoken, London, 1954), Chapter III; Holcombe, Victorian Ladies at Work, p. 11; Hutchins, Women in Modern Industry, p. 80.
8. Neff, Victorian Working Women, pp. 11-12; Hutchins, Women in Modern Industry, p. 75, Chapter III; Hammerton, Emigrant Gentlewomen, pp. 28-34.
9. M. Ebery and B. Preston, Domestic Service in Late Victorian and Edwardian England 1871 - 1914 (University of Reading, Reading, 1976), p. 18.
10. Ibid., p. 17.
11. S. Hogg, 'The Employment of Women in Great Britain 1891 - 1921', Unpublished D.Phil. Thesis, University of Oxford, 1964, p. 326a. See also C. Collet, 'The Collection and Utilisation of Official Statistics bearing on the extent and effects of the Industrial Employment of Women', Journal of the Royal Statistical Society, LXI, Part II, June 1898, pp. 219-70. For a discussion of the nature and importance of the service sector see, R. M. Hartwell, 'The Service Revolution: The Growth of Services in Modern Economy 1700 - 1914' in C. M. Cipolla (editor), Economic History of Europe, Volume 3: The Industrial Revolution (Fontana, London, 1977).
12. Hogg, 'Employment', p. 326a.
13. Branca, Women, pp. 51-2.
14. Ebery and Preston, Domestic Service, p. 2. See also S. Buckley, 'The Family and the Role of Women' in A. O'Day

(editor), The Edwardian Age: Conflict and Stability 1900 -
1914 (MacMillan, London, 1979), p. 137.

15. Ebery and Preston, Domestic Service, Tables 3a and
3b, p. 17, p. 21.

16. Ibid., p. 22, p. 112; P. E. Moulder, 'The General
Servant Problem', Westminster Review, CLX, August 1903; B. L.
Hutchins, 'Statistics of Women's Life and Employment', Journal
of the Royal Statistical Society, LXXII, Part II, 1909, p. 229;
'Domestic Service for Gentlewomen', British Association Meet-
ing, Bristol, 1875.

17. Cited in Ebery and Preston, Domestic Service, p. 22.

18. Ibid., pp.25-6.

19. Ibid., p. 88; Branca, Silent Sisterhood, pp. 34-6;
T. McBride, The Domestic Revolution: The Modernisation of
Household Service in England and France 1820 - 1920 (Croom
Helm, London, 1976), pp. 18-20, pp. 50-1; Banks, Prosperity,
pp. 70-85.

20. D. M. Barton, 'The Course of Women's Wages', Journal
of the Royal Statistical Society, (New Series), 82, (iv), July
1919, pp. 514-5; McBride, Domestic Revolution, pp. 49-69;
Ebery and Preston, Domestic Service, Chapter 4.

21. Ebery and Preston, Domestic Service, p. 85; McBride,
Domestic Revolution, Chapter 4.

22. Ebery and Preston, Domestic Service, p. 85; McBride,
Domestic Revolution, pp. 34-7, p. 75; M. Powell, Below Stairs
(Davies, London, 1968), pp. 4-5; P. Taylor, 'Daughters and
Mothers - maids and mistresses: Domestic Service between the
Wars' in J. Clarke et al (editors), Working Class Culture:
Studies in History and Theory (Hutchinson, London, 1974), p.
126; P. Horn, 'Domestic Service in Northampton 1830 - 1914',
Northampton Past and Present, 1973, pp. 267-73; L. Davidoff
Lockwood, 'Domestic Service and the Working Class Life Cycle',
Bulletin of the Society for the Study of Labour History, 26,
Spring 1973, p. 10; M. Thomas, 'Behind the Green Baize Door'
in N. Streatfield (editor), The Day Before Yesterday (Collins,
London, 1956), p. 80; J. Kitteringham, 'Country Work Girls in
Nineteenth-Century England' in R. Samuel (editor), Village
Life and Labour (Routledge and Kegan Paul, London, 1975), p.
132.

23. Ebery and Preston, Domestic Service, pp. 98-100;
McBride, Domestic Revolution, pp. 74-6; Branca, Women, p. 39
Horn, 'Northampton', p. 268; Thomas, 'Green Baize Door', p. 80.

24. W. Foley, A Child in the Forest (B.B.C., London,
1974) (1977 edition), p. 146; McBride, Domestic Revolution,
pp. 75-7; Ebery and Preston, Domestic Service, p. 85; Horn,
'Northampton', p. 268; Lockwood, 'Life Cycle', p. 12; Thomas,
'Green Baize Door', p. 82.

25. McBride, Domestic Revolution, Chapters 3 - 6; Branca,
Women, p. 39; Branca, Silent Sisterhood, pp. 56-7.

26. Ebery and Preston, Domestic Service, pp. 81-8;
McBride, Domestic Revolution, pp. 57-66; Branca, Women, p. 37;

W. T. Layton, 'The Changes in the Wages of Domestic Servants during 50 years', Journal of the Royal Statistical Society, LXXI, 1908, pp. 515-26; G. H. Wood, 'The Remuneration of the Woman Wage Earner Parts I and II', The English Woman, 7, (21), 1921 pp. 260-6, 8, (22), 1922, pp. 25-33; C. Booth, Life and Labour of the People in London (MacMillan, London, 1895), p. 133 et seq.

27. McBride, Domestic Revolution, p. 86.

28. Ibid., pp. 92-4.

29. Ibid., p. 120.

30. Taylor, 'Daughters and Mothers', p. 121; McBride, Domestic Revolution, Chapter 5, p. 121; Broom and Smith, 'Bridging Occupations', pp. 324-6; R. Strachey, Careers and Opportunities for Women (Faber and Faber, London, 1935), pp. 58-60. Lockwood advises, however, that "the claim of middle-class employers that experience of domestic service was the best training for working-class married life should ... be accepted with caution". 'Life Cycle', p. 11.

31. "Expansion of clerical opportunities for women really begins in the 1870's. The census figures for female commercial clerks in London go: 1857, 557; 1881, 2327; 1891, 6793; and other sources confirm that trend." Davin, 'Telegraphists', p. 9. See also, G. Anderson, 'The Social Economy of Late Victorian Clerks' in G. Crossick (editor), The Lower Middle Class in Britain 1870 - 1914 (Croom Helm, London, 1977), p. 127; G. Anderson, Victorian Clerks (Manchester University Press, Manchester, 1976), p. 2; Holcombe, Victorian Ladies at Work, Chapter VI, Appendix Table 4a, p. 210.

32. Holcombe, Victorian Ladies at Work, p. 141; Branca, Women, p. 55.

33. Holcombe, Victorian Ladies at Work, pp. 142-4; Anderson, 'Social Economy', p. 127; Davin, 'Telegraphists', p. 9; Strachey, Careers, p. 72; Buckley, 'Family', p. 136.

34. Holcombe, Victorian Ladies at Work, p. 142, pp.164-6; Anderson, Victorian Clerks, p. 12; Anderson, 'Social Economy', p. 127; Davin, 'Telegraphists', p. 7.

35. Anderson, 'Social Economy', p. 127. The opposite view is given by Hogg, 'Employment', p. 57, p. 71, and by contemporaries including Haynes, 'Occupations', p. 399; Lady Dilke et al (editors), Women's Work (Methuen, London, 1894), p. 42.

36. Holcombe, Victorian Ladies at Work, p. 144; Anderson, Victorian Clerks, p. 14.

37. Holcombe, Victorian Ladies at Work, pp. 144-6.

38. Ibid., Appendix Table 4a, p. 210.

39. Anderson, 'Social Economy', p. 127; Holcombe, Victorian Ladies at Work, p. 146. For a discussion of displacement see, Haynes, 'Occupations'.

40. Holcombe, Victorian Ladies at Work, p. 146.

41. Ibid., p. 146; Davin, 'Telegraphists', p. 8; Dilke, Women's Work, p. 44.

42. Holcombe, <u>Victorian Ladies at Work</u>, p. 146; Davin, 'Telegraphists', pp. 8-9.

43. Davin, 'Telegraphists', pp. 7-9.

44. Ibid., pp. 7-9.

45. Ibid., pp. 7-9.

46. Ibid., p. 9.

47. Ibid., p. 9.

48. Ibid., p. 9. See also, B. Hutchins, 'An Enquiry into the Wages and Hours of Work of Typists and Shorthand Writers', <u>Economic Journal</u>, XVI, September 1906, pp. 445-9.

49. Davin, 'Telegraphists', p. 9.

50. Ibid., p. 8.

51. Holcombe, <u>Victorian Ladies at Work</u>, pp.198-202.

52. Ibid., pp. 148-152; Strachey, <u>Careers</u>, pp. 59-60.

53. Davin, 'Telegraphists', p. 8; Holcombe, <u>Victorian Ladies at Work</u>, p. 178; H. Martindale, <u>Women Servants of the State 1870 - 1938: A History of Women in the Civil Service</u> (Allen and Unwin, London, 1938), pp. 147-9.

54. Holcombe, <u>Victorian Ladies at Work</u>, p.178, Mrs. Phillips (editor), <u>A Dictionary of Employments Open to Women</u> (Women's Institute, London, 1898), p. 112.

55. Holcombe, <u>Victorian Ladies at Work</u>, p. 178; M. Meredith, 'Women in the Civil Service: Part 1', <u>The English Woman</u>, 31, (1), July 1911, p. 38.

56. Meredith, 'Civil Service', p. 38; Holcombe, <u>Victorian Ladies at Work</u>, pp. 178-9.

57. Holcombe, <u>Victorian Ladies at Work,</u> pp. 156-62, pp. 179-93.

58. This Act was the first indication that the State was prepared to take on "the responsibility of placing an elementary education within reach of all". Part of that process was the creation of a new grade of teacher, the elementary school teacher. Holcombe, <u>Victorian Ladies at Work</u>, pp. 29-30; A. Tropp, <u>The School Teachers</u> (Heinemann, London, 1957), pp. 103-7; G. Partington, <u>Women Teachers in the 20th Century in England and Wales</u> (N. F. E. R., Windsor, 1976), p. 1; W. J. Reader, <u>Professional Men: The Rise of the Professional Classes in Nineteenth-Century England</u> (Weidenfeld and Nicolson, London, 1966), p. 181; Dilke, <u>Women's Work</u>, p. 8.

59. Holcombe, <u>Victorian Ladies at Work</u>, p. 34, p. 203; Partington, <u>Women Teachers</u>, pp. 1-3.

60. Partington, <u>Women Teachers</u>, p. 1; Holcombe, <u>Victorian Ladies at Work</u>, p. 35.

61. Partington, <u>Women Teachers</u>, p. 1.

62. Ibid., p. 1.

63. Holcombe, <u>Victorian Ladies at Work</u>, p. 36; Partington, <u>Women Teachers</u>, p. 1.

64. Partington, <u>Women Teachers</u>, p. 2; Holcombe, <u>Victorian Ladies at Work</u>, p. 36; Tropp, <u>School Teacher</u>, p. 187.

65. Partington, <u>Women Teachers</u>, p. 2.

66. A. Oram, 'The Employment of Women Teachers 1910 -

1938', Unpublished paper, University of Bristol, 1978, np.

67.   Partington, Women Teachers, pp. 3-4; Holcombe, Victorian Ladies at Work, p. 37; Tropp, School Teachers, p. 187.

68.   Holcombe, Victorian Ladies at Work, p. 37; Partington, Women Teachers, pp. 3-5.

69.   Holcombe, Victorian Ladies at Work, pp. 42-5; Partington, Women Teachers, pp. 8-9; Dilke, Women's Work, pp. 14-16; B. Webb, 'English Teachers and Their Professional Organisation', New Statesman Special Supplement, Vol. V, No. 129, September 1915, p. 2.

70.   Dilke, Women's Work.

71.   Ibid., p. 14. The Southampton School Board had the following salary scales (1899):

Head Teachers

	Class A £'s	Class B £'s	Class C £'s
Boys	180 - 240	150 - 200	140 - 160
Girls	100 - 150	100 - 130	90 - 120
Infants	100 - 150	100 - 130	90 - 120

Assistants

Boys	1st Assistant (Certificated and Trained)	£100 - 140
	2nd Assistant and Trained Assistant	£90 - 120
	Other Certificated Assistants	£70 - 100
Girls and Infants	1st Assistant	£70 - 100
	2nd Assistant	£70 - 90
	Others	£60 - 80
	Ex-Pupil Teachers	£40 - 50

Pupil Teachers

	Males £'s	Females £'s
1st Year	16	12
2nd Year	18	14
3rd Year	21	17
4th Year	25	21

All Pupil Teachers entering Training College receive an additional £10 per annum.

Source: Southampton School Board, Year Book 1899 (unpublished, Southampton Public Library).

72.   Tropp, School Teachers, p. 273.

73.   Holcombe, Victorian Ladies at Work, Chapter 3.

74.   Ibid., pp. 34-5. See also, Partington, Women Teachers, p. 98.

75.   Partington, Women Teachers, p.2. See also, J. Floud

and W. Scott, 'Recruitment to Teaching in England and Wales' in A. H. Halsey, J. Floud and A. Anderson (editors), Educa-tion, Economy and Society (Free Press, New York, 1961), pp. 527-44.

76. Partington, Women Teachers, p. 98.

77. F. Widdowson, 'Elementary Schoolmistresses 1900 - 1925', Unpublished paper, Oral History and Women's Work Con-ference, 1977. See also F. Widdowson, Going Up Into The Next Class: Women and Elementary Teacher Training 1840 - 1914 (Women's Research Resource Centre, London, 1980).

78. Widdowson, 'Elementary Schoolmistresses', pp. 2-3.

79. Ibid., p. 3.

80. Ibid., p. 2, p. 7. See also, Review of Conference in History Workshop, 4, Autumn 1977, pp. 234-5.

81. Holcombe, Victorian Ladies at Work, p. 37, pp. 66-7. See also, 'Teachers Registration Act', British Journal of Nursing, 23 October 1913, p. 33.

82. Holcombe, Victorian Ladies at Work, pp. 66-7.

83. Ibid.; p. 67.

84. Ibid., p. 68.

85. L. Stone, 'Literacy and Education in England 1640 - 1900', Past and Present, 42, 1969, p. 95; Partington, Women Teachers, p. 98.

86. Partington, Women Teachers, p. 96; Holcombe, Vic-torian Ladies at Work, p. 40.

87. Branca, Women, p. 11, p. 176; Partington, Women Teachers, pp. 95-9.

88. Shopwork also expanded as an area of women's employment in this period: see, Holcombe, Victorian Ladies at Work, pp. 103-40; Branca, Women, pp. 52-4; W. B. Whitaker, Victorian and Edwardian Shopworkers: The Struggle to obtain better conditions and a half-holiday (David and Charles, Newton Abbot, 1973).

Chapter 2

RECRUITMENT: SOCIAL AND OCCUPATIONAL MOBILITY

In 1905 Dr. Bedford Fenwick, one of the leading pro-Registrationists, told the Select Committee on the Registration of
Nurses that until the 1860's "there was practically no trained
nursing ... and no trained nurses." Those hospitals which did
exist tended to employ women as 'nurses' to keep the patients
and their surroundings clean and to give out medicines and
diets, women drawn mainly from the 'servant class'. Following
on from the Crimea War, and the influence of reformers like
Nightingale, a "better class" of women had entered the profession, leading to many improvements in the standards of care of
the hospital inmates.[1]
     At the same time, a writer of one nursing textbook, Miss
Voysey, informed her nurse readers (and potential nurse-recruits) that despite the influx of a few middle-class women
into the profession, nursing was "mixed as to rank", and more-
over, any discussion of the "social position" of nurses was
not "altogether a suitable subject" for inclusion in a nursing
textbook, since it was designed specifically to erase such
distinctions which might have existed by the promulgation of a
standard training programme.
     Despite Miss Voysey's reticence contemporaries, reformers
and recruits alike, were very concerned with the sort of womem
entering the new profession. It was essential to reform rhetoric that it be shown that the new nurses were markedly different from the old, pre-reform nurses of the Gamp age. At times
that concern was demonstrated by attempts to show that 'modern' nurses came from all ranks of society, as in the A to Z
list given to the Select Committee on the Metropolitan Hospitals by the Secretary of St. Bartholomew's Hospital, London
(1890).[3] On other occasions it took the form of the presenta-
tion of a prescriptive model, an ideal nurse, which sought to
define the nurse not in terms of 'class', but in terms of personal moral, physical, intellectual and emotional characteristics.[4] This latter approach to the discussion of the best
source of the nurse-recruit bowed a head towards the obvious
state of affairs, in which insufficient middle-class women took

up nursing despite the preferences of the reformers; it also allowed the profession to put itself above such material considerations as class, as well as allowing survivors of the rigorous training system to attack those who left the occupation in terms of individual failing, rather than present a potential critique of the hospital nursing regime as it then existed. We shall return to this theme in the discussion on training and socialisation: here we shall be concerned to re-examine the contemporary problem of recruitment to hospital nurse training. Five major questions will be addressed in order to better understand the structure of hospital nursing between 1881 - 1914: what were the geographical origins of the recruits?; did recruits work before taking up nurse-training?; why did women choose nursing?; how were women recruited to individual hospitals?, and how were the entrants selected from those who had applied to train?

The geography of recruitment
There is little in contemporary nursing sources to indicate where nurses lived prior to training. Miss Stansfield, an Assistant Inspector of the Poor Law in London, spoke of the "usefulness" of Scotch nurses, and like many others, of the numbers of girls who came from a farming background in this period.[5] Some matrons refused to take recruits from the immediate environs of the hospital, and given the frequency with which hospitals had sprung up in the poorest areas of most cities and towns, this may not be too surprising.[6] However, where recruits came from was intricately bound up in contemporary nursing ideology with recruiting the 'better class' of women: for example, either the harsh life of a nurse required her to be strong, and hence perhaps used to a rural lifestyle, or the reputation of a hospital for its training was such that it could recruit from anywhere in the kingdom.

Data from the sample hospitals about geographical mobility (Table 2.1) tend to conform to generally accepted patterns of female migration during the nineteenth-century.[7] In summary, women in the period tended to be more migratory than men, with a "constant movement" from rural to urban areas which for the most part was of short-distance, with long-distance migration being preferentially towards "one of the great centres of commerce and industry".[8]

The data show a distinction in geographical recruitment patterns between voluntary and Poor Law sectors in two important aspects; first in the proportion of local women recruited, and second, in the proportion of women recruited from Ireland, Scotland and Wales. Both aspects may have more to do with the role specific towns played in overall migration patterns than deliberate choice either by the women or by the recruiting hospitals. The number of women recruited from Ireland and Wales in particular, and to some extent also from Scotland, illustrates the way in which such migrants moved considerable

Table 2.1: Geographical Origins of Recruits to Nursing 1881 - 1921 [a]

Hospitals	Town	(miles) 0-20m	20-50m	50-150m	150+m	Ire-land	Scot-land	Wales	Other	Totals
Southampton Poor Law Infirmary	100	48	22	51	34	36	4	29	1	325
Portsmouth Poor Law Infirmary	228	33	15	39	15	12	1	11	-	354
Leeds Poor Law Infirmary	55	55	57	85	10	32	16	27	3	340
Salisbury General Infirmary	37	35	86	91	25	14	7	12	10	317
Winchester Royal Hants Infirmary	17	124	39	129	23	20	9	14	6	381
Totals	437	295	219	395	107	114	37	93	20	1717

Source: Hospital Records (unpublished)

a. For actual dates of individual hospitals see, Chapter 1, above.

distances but towards the major centres, rather than the small market towns and rural communities.[9]

Given the instances of claims by contemporaries that women chose particular hospitals for the prestige which training in them offered,[10] and the relatively small nursing population involved, it would be pertinent to look .at other more occupationally-specific factors which determined patterns of nurse-recruitment. Indeed, to relate nurse-recruitment solely to general patterns of female migration might assume that nursing was the object of that movement, and that other alternative work experiences were not considered by the women. We need to take account of motives, alternative occupations and other variables in order to fully explain nurse-recruitment in this first generation of hospital training.

Occupational change to nursing

As we have noted (Chapter 1), contemporaries assumed and at times appeared to demand that recruits to training came fresh or only via approved intermediate work experiences. On other occasions commentators referred to recruits as coming from the "servant class",[11] particularly, although not exclusively, in the Poor Law Sector. How far they were correct or justified in these assertions may be judged from an analysis of the nurses' registers kept by the sample hospitals, which listed (although not with the precision we would like) the previous work experiences of the recruits. Using that data we can learn whether nursing was a first work choice for a majority of contemporary nurses, or whether nursing, like domestic service,[12] offered some women the opportunity not only for geographical but for social mobility, and was in consequence merely a stepping-stone in a series of work choices.

The sample data (Table 2.2) show clearly that while a proportion of all nurse-recruits had had no (acknowledged) previous work experience prior to entry, a majority (71%) had actually held paid employment before nurse training. Superficially, the significant minority of recruits who had no previous work record (Nil) lends support for contemporary claims that recruits came to nursing as a first deliberate choice. Closer analysis, however, reveals reservations about the overall size of this group and in consequence, contemporary claims about the ideal nurse recruit. First, the actual entries in the records are at times ambiguous - while at the point of entry the recruit might have been 'unoccupied' it is clear in a number of cases that this statement was not intended to characterise the entire work record of the entrant. Second, some of these 'previously unoccupied' women had contributed to the family economy without receiving wages. For example, one woman who said she had not worked before nursing had in fact helped her father in his job as a small town newspaper editor in Canada. Another had "brought up my mother's children because she was blind after her first childbirth", and had done

Table 2.2: Previous Work Experiences of Recruits to Nurse Training 1881 - 1921 [a]

	M.R.I. (Manchester)	The London	Leeds	Portsmouth	Totals
Nil	478	1240	103	147	1968
Nursing	658	1161	131	87	2037
Domestic Service	351	1290	81	42	1664
Clerical and Commercial	66	224	10	28	328
Clothing and Textiles	22	84	19	18	143
Shopwork	29	104	16	28	177
Education	85	228	7	3	323
Warwork, Miscellaneous	7	123	3	14	147
Totals	1696	4454	370	367	6887

Source: Hospital Records (Unpublished)

a. For actual dates of individual hospitals see, Chapter 1, above

all the myriad of household duties common to women of her background.[13]

The only recruits for which we can be sure of the accuracy of the unoccupied category are those under-21 year old entrants in the final years of the sample, who appear to have come almost straight from secondary school as the age of entry to nursing was drastically reduced to meet the acute shortage of recruits in those years and those widows and few single women aged over 30 years of age who had either been housewives for most of their adult life or housekeepers to relatives for the same time. In total, these two groups made up only 1C.6% of all recruits in the sample. Even this revised figure fails to fit the ideal type referred to earlier.

The data show that there was a redistribution of female labour away from such occupations as clerical and commercial work, clothing and textile work, teaching and shopkeeping, and into nursing. However, this entire group of recruits formed only 14% of the total recruits in the sample although the annual rate at which, in particular, clerical and commercial recruits joined increased as the period developed.[14] Such women had potentially much to offer nursing. The relatively high educational standards required by the employers of such workers and the possibility of formal training, as in the case of telephonists, added to the social prestige which this type of work offered to women. The demand and supply of secretarial courses, especially in London, demonstrate not only the growing need for such 'trained' office and clerical workers, but also the eagerness on the part of women to choose it as a job. For some women there was the possibility, as in shopwork, of direct consumer or client relationships, and the dress, manners and bearing which the situation required of the worker acted to reinforce the prestige of some areas of clerical and commercial work. Added to these work advantages was the likelihood of extending social contacts, particularly among men, and hence increasing the chances of making a 'better' marriage.[15]

Actual work conditions for most women in such jobs seldom matched their expectations. For many, clerical work meant the large commercial office and the virtual anonymity of working in a large group of similarly placed women: for others it meant the cage of a cash-desk, often perched high above the sales area of a store or large shop, seldom coming into contact with fellow workers, let alone potential social contacts amongst the customers. For most, such work meant long hours, poor wages and in some instances a system of living-in and a toll of fines for 'misdemeanours'.[16] It is, therefore, no surprise that a proportion of recruits to hospital nursing came from the ranks of such workers, although whether they were consciously rejecting one controlled community for another, or saw in nursing, despite its disciplined regime, a justification for control over their lives through service to others, is unclear.

The appearance of one group of women in this section of
the recruit sample seems to argue that nursing was positively
recruiting among women with higher qualifications than many,
i.e. teaching. However, at least 25% of these recruits were
teachers of music, drama or physical-culture, demand for whom
tended to depend on fashion rather than on educational needs
or developments. The few (less than 20) secondary school teachers who appear in this sample may have entered nursing not
so much positively as in response to competition for posts
with male teachers in the higher sector of education.

The other 'teachers' in the recruit sample (243 in total)
were almost always uncertificated, unqualified or pupil-tea-
chers, with a few private teachers included. Such women were
experiencing increased competition for jobs in the elementary
sector, not so much from men, but more from the numbers of
trained women teachers entering the field.[17] The general conclusion about the presence of many of these women in the recruit sample is that they came less because nursing set out to
attract them, and more because they were being excluded from
their own occupational groups. While they may have had qualities which nursing needed, including experience of some degree
of work-discipline, it is likely that nursing drew them in because it offered a further chance of entering a new, and hence
as yet 'open' occupation, in which they could as easily acquire a training and qualification as any other recruit.[18]

Most recruits came not from these areas of work, however,
but from two major sectors of employment, domestic service and
other areas of nursing itself. The first group are consistent
with contemporary observations of nursing, but the latter are
almost totally absent from both contemporary and secondary
literature on nursing development. Such recruits made up over
55% of all recruits in the sample, 2037 out of the 6887 recruits.

Domestic service was an amorphous group whose prime common experience was the provision of "a personal service for
their master or mistress" or employer.[19] With the increasing
specialisation towards the end of the nineteenth-century, this
service could be provided within the limits of the home - indoor servants -, within the confines of the employers' pro-
perty but outside of the living accommodation - outdoor servants - or in communal or business settings, such as offices,
laundries, hairdressing salons, etc. - auxilliary domestic
servants.[20]

All categories of contemporary service are shown in the
recruit data: however, as Table 2.3 clearly demonstrates, most
recruits from this sector came from the ranks of indoor servants with those servants who provided their labour at the top
of the servant hierarchy or whose work directly substituted for
one or more of the personal roles of the employer, for example,
the rearing or socialization of children, being most prominent
in the sample.

Table 2.3: Recruits to Nursing with Domestic Service Experience, 1881 – 1921, to selected hospitals[a]

Hospital	All Grades	Cooks H/Keepers	General Servant	House + Parlour Maid	Ladys Maid	Mothers Help/ Childs Nurse	Governess	Companion	Others
Leeds	81	8	20	13	5	3	18	10	4
Portsmouth	42	1	6	6	1	12	14	-	2
Manchester	351	49	94	23	19	53	87	18	8
The London	1290	80	71	100	66	535	179	156	103
Totals	1764	138	191	142	91	603	298	184	117

Source: Hospital Records (Unpublished)

a. For actual dates of individual hospitals, see, Chapter 1, above.

While all grades appear throughout the years of the sample, recruits from the lower echelons of indoor service, in particular general servants, parlour- and housemaids, tend to be concentrated in the years 1881 - 1901, or more appositely in the first years of probationer training (even when that occurred after 1901 as in the case of Portsmouth Poor Law Hospital). At this distance it is difficult to explain this distribution satisfactorily; however, it is likely that the links between nursing and domestic service - hygiene, cleaning and household management - made such recruits the 'new brooms' of nursing in the early years of training.

Hospital nurse recruits did come from domestic service, then, as contemporaries claimed, and some lamented: however, even more came from within the heterogeneous occupation itself (Table 2.2). Such women formed two distinct groups; first, those who were already in the general hospital sector, and wished to change hospital for one reason or another; and second, women working as nurses outside of the general hospitals as private nurses, maternity and cottage nurses, fever nurses, mental nurses and children's hospital nurses etc. (Table 2.4).

Those nurses already in the general sector moved for a variety of reasons, including a dislike of a particular hospital or style of discipline; personal disagreement with a matron, ill-health or a wish to be nearer home. A few appear to have been undecided about where to work or train as nurses, and a small group moved because they found themselves in the 'wrong' sort of hospital, i.e. Poor Law rather than voluntary. [21]

Just over half of this type of recruit (1022, 50.2% of 'nurse' entrants) came from the specialised branches of nursing, both institutional and non-institutional, from women without general hospital training or even any form of hospital experience, let alone experience of training in them. Competition for patients, and hence survival, both personal and occupational, lay behind this trend, and the experience of many non-general nurses may be typified by what was happening to maternity and to private nurses.

The London Obstetrical Society had offered its certificate to women passing their external examinations since the late 1890's; many hospitals provided their nurses with the opportunity to acquire midwifery experience, and the specialised women and children's hospitals gave from 3 - 6 months training in midwifery and maternity nursing. After the 1902 Midwives Act, the Central Midwives Board certificated women as midwives after a prescribed training at a 'recognised' institution. The occupational struggle between the man-midwives, the doctors and the nurse-midwives accounts for some women seeking alternative nursing work in the early twentieth-century.[22] It is also probable that the increasing use of maternity beds and more impotantly the provision of maternity nurses by the voluntary hospitals' private staffs offered a burden of competition that

Table 2.4: Nurse-Recruits with experience of Nursing, 1881 - 1921 to selected hospitals [a]

Hospital	Hospital Nursing [b]	Special Hospital Nursing [c]	Maternity, Cottage, District Nursing [d]	Private Nursing [e]	Others [f]	Totals
Leeds	94	8	7	4	18	131
Portsmouth	34	12	7	5	29	87
Manchester	411	144	20	10	73	658
The London	476	277	150	114	144	1161
Totals	1015	441	184	133	264	2037

Source: Hospital Records (Unpublished)

a. For actual dates of individual hospitals, see Chapter 1
b. Includes those returned as "Nurse"; "Probationer"; "Nursing"
c. Fever nurses; Children's Hospital nurses; Women's Hospital nurses
d. Midwives and women holding Central Midwives Board or London Obstetrical Society certificates
e. Lady nurses; private nurses; Nursing Association and Institute nurses
f. Mental nurses; convalescent nurses; highly specialized nursing, e.g. Home for Cripples, and Volunteer Aid Detachment nurses.

many such women were unable to bear.[23] Those maternity and midwife nurses who could not compete faced the prospect of joining an agency and losing their independence to choose clients; applying to the private staff of a voluntary hospital and losing control over their work and social lives, or trying to obtain a general hospital training in order to be able to supplement maternity work with general nursing work outside of the hospitals.

The falling fortunes of the private nurse, although delayed temporarily by a boom in the demand for care in the home by the middle and upper-classes, as with all forms of contemporary service, were brought about by two factors. First, the growth of hospital provision in general:[24] while there was an initial reluctance for the class most likely to employ private nurses to enter hospitals for care, this was quickly overcome as developments in the standard of care and the increasing cheapness of in-patient care (even if on the private wards of the voluntary hospitals) compared to the cost of hiring personal nurses made the hospitals more attractive to this class.[25]

Second, those hospitals which began to attract the potential employers of private nurses, i.e. the voluntary hospitals, also began to set up and manage staffs of private nurses. These nurses, with the hospital's name to recommend them as 'trained' and the hospital's own doctors determining the care needed by the patients in their homes, tended to exclude many of the existing private, and often 'untrained', nurses who had little but their own local reputations to recommend them to clients.[26] Since many of the nurses training in the voluntary hospitals worked on the private staff during or immediately after training, or were recruited by the matrons directly after training to be private nurses, there was no shortage of 'trained' private nurses available from these hospitals. The value of such nurses was widely known, if not always acknowledged; not only did they carry out a sort of publicity function for the good name of the hospital, they also brought in valuable revenue at a time when the voluntary hospitals were facing acute financial crises.[27] At the London Hospital, for example, Burdett estimated that after all deductions the private staff of that hospital netted £4,000 per annum,[28] and the private staff nurses were rarely paid a full salary - "the hospital was getting £3 a week for me on the private staff while I was only getting a small salary. That was the way I paid for it, my training."[29] As Burdett succintly put it, the hospitals were taking from the new generation of nurses "with both hands".[30]

Individual nurses came to general training from a variety of backgrounds and from all over the kingdom, some from beyond. However, clear patterns seem to emerge from the sample which if not directly challenging contemporary stereotypes, go some way to making them more illuminating in a discussion of occupa-

tional recruitment. Of most significance is the previous work
experience of recruits to general training, and the high proportion of non-general but practising nurses in the sample.
While structural changes in the occupation, as described
above, explain why this group figures so prominently in nurse
recruitment, we shall need to look more closely at why women
chose to take up general nursing to better understand the process by which general nursing was coming to establish itself
as the ideologically dominant sector of the occupation.

Why did women choose nursing?

Among other considerations the choice of a career or an area
of work implies an awareness of choice; the existence of potential alternatives; the ability or opportunity for making a
choice, and the personal capacity of achieving that selection.
31 Indeed, the possibility of a choice between work and non-
work has to be included, and would be most important in a
study of the motivation and recruitment process as it affected
a section of the nursing elite - women like Nightingale, Fenwick, Jones and other members of the middle-classes.

While it was the case that for men the restrictions on
the choice of work were rarely "so extreme that the individual
(could) be said to be in a 'no-work' situation",32 an examination of the occupation tables of the relevant census shows
that many contemporary women, and indeed men, were restricted
in the choice of work, especially when local and regional
variations are considered. Much contemporary employment was
either rural- or urban-specific (agriculture or manufacture);
sex-specific (e.g. law); age-specific, or a combination of all
three. Consequently, even before other considerations are discussed, much of the potential choice of work had been eradica-
ted from most peoples' lives.33

Within even this narrower range of occupational choice,
however, many women did exercise or attempt to exercise some
selectivity about the type or grade of work they were to follow, even if all this meant was that they changed jobs frequently in their early work years. In domestic service this
constant change was not only an attempt at betterment and the
acquisition of 'skills', but also an attempt to find the
"better positions", if not the ideal one.34 Young women were
accustomed, then, to frequent changes of work either within
the same occupation or, as in the case of some nurse recruits,
to alternatiave areas of work; these examples show this common
tendency among nurse recruits -

> First I went to Boots to train; then I started train-
> ing as a hairdresser, which was useless, and my sister
> had started at a small fever hospital, and as soon as
> she went, you know, to get away from sharing beds and
> so on, I pressed to be a nurse.

My sister had got me apprenticed to a milliners in
Portsmouth when I was 16 but I wasn't very keen on
it. So I came home and looked after the other six
children. I was 21 when I applied for probationer
training at St. Mary's.

I was one of five and they, my parents, were not
very ambitious for me, and I was very lucky to get
into a hospital. I'd been in a chemist's and then
I went to train as a dispenser.[35]

As the last example suggests, not only did the women themselves select their work, their parents and family might also
play an important albeit negative part in the process. Three
typical parental/family attitudes emerge from the remarks of
interviewed nurses. First, an outright and often effusive acceptance of nursing as work for the girl - "mother didn't mind,
oh! mother was content"; "my father was very keen ... he was
very pleased when I wanted to train." Second, the family were
sceptical about the choice, could the girl stand the life of a
nurse, did she have the resolve to do the work? Usually, this
attitude pointed out the "dreadful things" nurses had to do,
bedpans and so on; occasionally, it was the harshness of the
discipline which caused the family's scepticism - "you'll be
home the first week because someone said something to you".
Finally, some parents and families disapproved either of nursing or of any sort of work for the girl :-

My mother wouldn't let me go into a shop, it wasn't
done, and she wouldn't let me go in for higher education, which I would have done to become a teacher but
she didn't see the point.[36]

None of these women chose nursing as a first choice of
work; indeed, most, as in the case of the recruit sample, came
to nursing after other work experiences. What was it that put
the idea of nursing as work into their minds, apart from those
having a close relative who was already in the occupation?
What did nursing appear to offer them which perhaps other jobs
did not?
Ginsberg has drawn our attention to the relationships between occupational choice and the stages of maturity of the
individual.[37] Three distinct patterns of choice, "fantasy
choice", "tentative choice" and "realistic choice", in career
decisions correspond to specific stages in the maturation of
the person, i.e. early childhood and pubescence; early adolescence; and maturity itself. Whether or not work choice depends
upon such a process it is possible to see similar patterns in
the responses by nurses to questioning about why they had
chosen nursing as a career. Indeed Burdett began one of his
books on nursing with a fantasy-like explanation for the popularity of nursing -

Every boy in his teens wants to be a sailor; every
girl in her teens wants to be a nurse. The boy probably outgrows the romantic period and turns to other
thoughts during his college life; but the girl, unless
she contracts an early marriage, casts longing eyes on
the hospital world, whenever her home becomes dull and
dances fail to satisfy her mind.[38]

The romance of nursing, generated in part in popular fiction, came also from the everyday world of some girls. One
such woman saw a uniformed nurse arrive in her village with a
doctor to care for a sick 'lady'; aged about twelve she
thought "how wonderful it (was) to work with a doctor, and to
be able to cure the lady".[39] Other girls played with dolls and
were encouraged by their families to play at 'doctors and
nurses'.

I'd always wanted to be a nurse. As a child I'd
always hated dolls and the only reason I used them
for was ward beds in a row. I'd never seen a hospital and I used to line them up in a row, and my
father would come and prescribe for them. I don't
know where I got the idea from, it was instinct.
I'd never been in a hospital; I didn't get the idea
from books. I used to do all sorts of things to
those dolls. So I'd always wanted to be a nurse.[40]

The gender stereotyping of play and of nursing pushed
over into the dreams of the adolescent girl. In her autobiography, E. C. Laurence wrote to a friend of the romantic notion of winning a medal in the service of the Queen: since
"none of the professions in which my brothers were distinguish-
ing themselves would be open to me", (i.e. military service),
Laurence decided to become a nurse, and to "try to win the
Royal Red Cross".[41] Even when the opportunity for medals passed, with the end of the Boer Wars, she still determined to be
a nurse, perhaps like a much later nurse, Joan Markham, finding herself trapped into the decision by the impetuosity of
youth. "I'm going to be a nurse! The family may have been
surprised at my decision, but they were not half so surprised
as I was. It was an off the cuff remark that had received no
consideration, but as I heard myself make the announcement, the
possibility became a probability."[42]

For those women who saw nursing only in a tentative light,
as perhaps a suitable choice for them but one which they were
not entirely happy about making, the choice was often between
the boredom of home life and some vague notion of the need for
a 'vocation' for nursing. "I never thought about my job really",
one elderly nurse recalled, "my parents wanted me to go into a
shop, materials and that sort of thing, but I wasn't keen on
it; no, I didn't do anything, I was just at home helping out

generally." The determining factor in this woman's life was her experiences as a V.A.D. in the First World War, when the fantasy element combined with the boredom of her pre-war home to push her into making the decision to train.[43]

Other women, often with several years of work experience behind them, chose to train as general nurses either as an end in itself or as a means to an end, and usually after consider-able thought about the decision. For some the physical acti-vity of nursing made it appear more attractive than the seden-tary jobs such as clerical or civil service work; for others the potential for infinite variety, of patients and tasks, was the deciding factor. "I looked around the railway office and there was a lot of spinsters there in the supervisory jobs, and I thought, fancy coming here, year in, year out, suppos-ing: year in, year out, just in this thing."[44] And, as this last example suggests, there was always the possibility of making a marriage, with a doctor or with a patient. For a few, perhaps a more realistic few, nursing offered them a chance to acquire a skill which could be used to provide for them in their old, and unmarried years. One woman wanted to run a home for homeless children, and decided that she just "had to get my nursing certificate"; her original intentions for entering nursing were forgotten, however, when she became a ward sister and then an assistant matron, but she was remembered by her matron in later years for the strength of her original resolve and ambition - "she used to tease me about it afterwards. She said, "You did know what you wanted."[45]

How were women recruited?
Having decided to become a nurse, no matter how that decision was arrived at, the girl was faced with the immediate problem of how and where? She had to find a hospital willing to employ her, and more and more importantly, to train her and give her a certificate as a trained nurse.

It was the proud boast of many matrons that they always had a waiting-list of girls queueing up to train in their hos-pital. The impression generated is of too many applicants chasing too few vacancies, and only the 'best' being chosen. Abel-Smith recently reiterated this contemporary rhetoric -

> In so far as it was the object of the nursing reform movement to attract suitable women to the hospital this was achieved. As time went on the first trickle of timorous pupils was followed by a steady and suf-ficient stream of suitable candidates. Later still the stream became a torrent. Many hospitals had more applicants than they could accommodate.[46]

The Annual Return of the Poplar and Stepney Sick Asylum for 1902 reported that 76 women had applied to be probationers there, with 23 appointed and another 10 kept "on the books,

awaiting appointment" when a vacancy occurred. The Hon.
Sidney Holland, Hon. Secretary to the London Hospital, told a
Select Committee that while not all applicants were of the
"right class", at the London Hospital there was "no shortage
of applicants in actual numbers".[47] Burdett, a stickler for
figures, handed in a paper to the same Committee, which
showed that there were at least 18 applicants for every
vacancy for probationer training in the voluntary general and
Poor Law hospitals.[48] At this time Guy's Hospital was said to
have 2,000 applications for 140 annual vacancies; Liverpool
Royal Infirmary 900 for 30 vacancies, and Leeds General Infirmary 400 applicants for 20 vacancies. Even excluding entirely 'unsuitable candidates', one leading nurse claimed
that many women were having to wait one, two or even more
years before finding a vacancy at one of these hospitals.[49]

A more realistic and cautionary note was sounded by Eva
Luckes, the matron of the London Hospital, a leading anti-
registrationist; "as to the number of candidates from which
you may choose, the number has been greatly exaggerated. The
candidates write round to 4 or 5 hospitals so as to be able
to take their choice of a vacancy. That number that has been
given does not represent the number of women who really wish
to become nurses."[50] This multiple application practice was
an extensive and long-standing feature of nurse recruitment.
In 1909 in a letter to a nursing journal an "Applicant" said
she had applied to four hospitals simultaneously for training,
while in 1914 one matron proposed setting up a "blacklist" to
be published weekly in the nursing press, to include the names
of women who, having applied to several hospitals for admission, failed to turn up after being offered posts in them.[51]

While an average of three or four applicants for each
actual post would seem a fairer estimate of the popularity of
nurse training, this only applied to the larger and more well-
known hospitals. In some of the smaller Poor Law and voluntary
training hospitals there was a rather more constant problem of
recruiting sufficient nurses, trained and untrained. At the
Royal South Hants Infirmary the matron was given permission by
the Management Committee in 1890 to advertise for staff in the
national press, and in 1919 the continued problem of lack of
recruits forced the then matron, Miss Jenkins, to write to the
Committee complaining of her lack of success in finding probationers and asking that the nurses' salaries be raised in
order to attract more women to the hospital.[52] Overall, then,
recruitment of suitable numbers, and of suitable women, was
not as easy as some nurse leaders suggested; further evidence
for this situation of scarcity of recruits comes from the discussion of the discipline system in nursing. If women were
truly queueing up in their thousands to train, why were so few
of them dismissed for breaches of the discipline codes? Wil-
liam Rathbone, reformer, businessman and Chairman of Brownlow
Hill Infirmary, Liverpool, might have very well urged the

matrons to dismiss more of the 'unsuitable' nurses,[53] but most
matrons were well aware that there was not an endless supply,
and anyway those who might be on a waiting list could turn out
just as bad, and cost the hospital and nursing staff as much
time and money and patience as they had already expended on
the incumbent. We shall return to this theme in the discussion
over the trial period and "wastage" during training; here it
may serve to remind us that many contemporary nursing statements were for public consumption, rather than for accurately
describing the nursing scene.

As the South Hants experience shows, the would-be nurse
could consult either the specialised literature which carried
advertisements for individual hospitals requiring probationers,
or the local or national press: occasionally, the girl might
learn about a vacancy or possibility of training through more
direct, word-of-mouth contacts. There are examples of the influence of friends writing to each other and discussing nursing, particular hospitals or training schools, there is also
evidence of the more direct recommendation of a woman by a
friend who was already a nurse to a particular hospital matron:-

17/6/07   Miss S. from Warminster: occupation -
           miniature painter; recommended by Nurse E.
 4/9/07   Miss T. from Woolwich; occupation - First
           assistant nurse; recommended by Nurse T.
30/1/09   Miss S. from Sydenham; occupation - Assis-
           tant home nurse; recommended by Nurse E.[54]

The personal recommendation of a woman for training had
more force if it came from a person of some social standing,
for example, a local business-man, a member of the local Board
of Guardians, a priest, or a subscriber of importance to a
voluntary hospital. There were disadvantages in this informal
method of recruitment, in particular for any woman not aware
of the distinctions between Poor Law and voluntary sectors and
some undoubtedly either ended up in the wrong type of training
or were forced to move once the mistake was realised.

Less confusion arose if the prospective nurse made use of
the advertisements in the press or the advice given in the
many contemporary guides to careers, most of which gave details of the type and size of the hospital, salaries and some
outline of the conditions of service to be expected.[55] The
guides to employment,[56] those in particular like Burdett's
Hospital Annual which were for nurses only, were not strictly
advertising vacancies, but rather opportunities: however, the
fact that many hospitals felt it necessary to be included in
such publications, together with the explicit advertisements
in such journals as The Lancet, The Lady, The Poor Law Officers Journal or The British Medical Journal, once again belies
the confident contemporary assertions about the numbers of

women desperate to train.

The woman who was able to and actively sought a career choice was faced, then, with a wide range of literature about nursing. But however much this material was read, actual recruits applied to specific hospitals in response to known vacancies as much as in a general attempt to get on a waiting-list. This is not only born out by the extensive use by matrons of advertisements for staff, but by the numbers of recruits who came from the hospital-area, suggesting a local acquaintance with the hospital and the staff levels.

The nationality and religious persuasion of the matron, on occasion both, could also be a factor in deciding which hospital to choose, in particular for recruits from outside of England -

> As a matter of fact, at this hospital the matron was a converted 'RC' and she filled the hospital with girls from Ireland, from convents and convent schools, you know. I didn't know 'til afterwards, they used to call it the 'Irish Hospital'. That was the last place my mother would have wanted me to go. She (matron) got them through the priests. They were Irish farm girls and girls from convents, you know, all mad keen to get to London, they thought it was wonderful.[57]

If some of the matrons were correct in their assessment of the number of applicants coming forward, how did the individual matron pick suitable candidates? Most applicants began by writing to the matron of the hospital of their choice, although some women applied in person, suggesting that local recruitment was not so unusual. The usual response to the inquiry about training was the sending of an application form to be completed in the woman's own hand, and normally to be returned with at least two testimonials. On occasion, a photograph of the candidate was also required.

References were generally accepted as bona fide if they were sent with the form: where testimonials were sought after the interview problems might arise in obtaining them from the previous employer, which may have reflected unfairly on the candidate.

The application form not only provided information about the recruit, but was also a means of assessing the literacy and education level of the woman. The manner and the handwriting were important indicators of suitability to nurse -

> 6/9/05 Miss M. from Greenwich; aged 22; nil occupation; 'Writes a very bad hand and does not appear to have been very well educated'
> 17/3/17 Miss T. from Cork; aged 22; housekeeper; 'Application form badly filled in'.[58]

The photograph of the applicant, where asked for, appears somewhat innocuous, making it easier for the matron to recognise the applicant when she arrived for interview or to begin the trial period before actual training: "I did it all by letter; I had to send a photo, I remember, because when I got there she said I didn't look a bit like my photo."[59] There is some reason to argue that the photograph played a more important part in the actual selection process. Within the nursing context, it was part of the matron's role to be able to recognise on sight, or in this case from a photograph, whether an applicant would make a suitable nurse.[60] The ability of the matron to recognize a suitable recruit in this way coincided with the tendency to cede to her responsibility for the recruitment, management and training of probationers, as her authority within the hospital and the nursing world rose. Inevitably, this process tended towards positive recruitment of like-minded recruits, women acceptable to the leadership rather than from a true cross-section of the female population.

The manner in which the application had been made, the handwriting, the photograph and perhaps the previous work experiences of the applicant weighed most heavily in the matron's mind when making her decision. The on-sight recognition of suitability added to this preliminary 'weeding-out' process to diminish the importance of the first interview in contemporary nursing management practice. For many applicants, however, the interview with the matron or Management Committee was still a daunting affair, although as one woman found out, it could turn out to be a test of ability to fit in with a closed community, rather than of academic suitability -

My interview was with the Matron who was very much St. Thomas' trained and an A.R.R.C. She appeared to be much more interested in my social life and then proceeded to find out if I had any knowledge of Art, and could I recognise any of the pictures? I could and I did.[61]

The interview, crude though it was even in terms of contemporary management techniques, was not the final hurdle the would-be nurse had to face in order to get into training. There remained the trial period, lasting from one to three months, during which the new probationer was closely observed and which allowed for either party to withdraw from the training commitment.

The trial period was in almost universal use at this time and applied as much to the smaller and more specialised hospitals as to the larger training schools. In a few, the month(s) spent 'on trial' counted as part of the total training period:[62] for the majority of nurses it was in addition to the 2, 3 or 4 years of training. It could be unpaid and indeed very costly for the applicant who might have to supply some or all of her uniform for the trial period. Some women in the voluntary hospitals paid an "entrance fee", a "training fee" or "premium", which was returned in some cases if the woman remained to train, or was subject to deductions or complete forfeit if the woman left during this period or without "reasonable notice" during the actual training years.[63]

The precise financial burden of the trial period is difficult to assess; there is no way, for example, of deciding how many left during the trial through lack of income, and it is possible that the provision of board, lodging and other emoluments reduced the overall financial cost to individuals. For some women the entrance fee forced them into the Poor Law sector,[64] for others it was part of the status of voluntary hospital training -

> I went to the West Middlesex; well, of course, you
> hadn't to pay anything, it was a Poor Law and every-
> thing ... Later I went to U.C.H. and, of course, my
> father had to pay £50 there.[65]

While the prospect of a premium or of no income for some time might have excluded a few women from nursing, or from their preferred type of hospital, the recruit sample suggests that most of the recruits were in work which could provide some opportunity of accumulating savings, even in domestic service. The women who might have found this period particularly hard were those who were used to sending all or most of their earnings back to their families, a common enough practice for working women at this time.

The trial period was in extensive use throughout our period, and as a stage in the recruitment process was used by both hospital and recruit as a final test of suitability. The turn-over rate was high, on average 22% of entrants left in the trial period,[66] justifying its existence. As the records of Manchester Royal Infirmary note

> January 1908 - December 1921: 975 probationers.
> 43 not strong enough to continue after having
> passed the doctor; 11 deaths; 130 left for other
> reasons; <u>200 left before completion of trial months,
> having felt the months too much of a trial, or been
> too much of a trial</u> (sic). (emphasis added)[67]

This relatively high 'failure rate' during the trial months was not only self-justificatory, it also calls into question the expected ability of the matron to recognise the right type of recruit: why was such an experienced nurse-manager so often wrong in her judgement?

Some women left for reasons consistent with the role assigned to the matron as the recruiter; for example, due to ill-health; because they were "wanted at home", or because the woman found herself in the wrong sort of hospital. The others left for reasons not so easily compatible with the matron's ability to recognise the best candidate on sight - some 'ran away' or were of "questionable character"; some failed the educational and nursing tests taken in the trial months, and a few gave up nursing all together having found that it did not 'suit them'. However, a distinction was made by the matron between acceptable reasons for leaving and those the hospital was not prepared to accept. Acceptable reasons were briefly listed in the records as "very promising candidate who was called home",; "wished to be nearer home"; or as "too delicate for training". Against the names of those women who left for unacceptable reasons were written often longer comments, such as "unsuitable for training, not interested in her work and too free with soldier patients"; "most unsuitable for a nurse; conduct unsatisfactory. Appears to have a mania for running up bills which she cannot pay; found smacking a child and altogether bad tempered"; or the worst reason of all, "did not like nursing, she said it was unpleasant."[68]

It does not matter, especially at this distance, whether such statements are true or not: rather it is the way in which such distinctions are made in the records which is more relevant.[69] The almost weekly departures[70] of one or several recruits were seen not as criticisms of the selection process, and still less of the matron's role in it, but were presented in terms which indicted the individual rather than the occupation or even the hospital. That is to say, having accepted a degree of 'wastage' during the trial months - or else why have a trial at all - the fault or reason for withdrawal was laid at the feet of the individual recruit. She was either emotionally inadequate ("too neurotic"); morally unsound ("inclined to flirt with male patients"); educationally backward ("too lazy to study"), and so on. The matron and the selection process were vindicated by those who fell; even those women who might have been guileless enough to trick the matron initially could not survive the rigours of the nurse's life. The trial period found even these women out.

Contemporary occupational concern about the type of woman who would make the best nurse, linked as it was to the controversy over State Registration, has tended to obscure a full understanding of why and how women made the choice to nurse. In their attempts to exclude specific groups from entry to nursing or from existing areas of nursing practice, nursing reformers and matrons put forward prescriptive models of the ideal nurse, some of which survive into recent literature. In attempting to select, hospital nursing was in effect creating a hierarchy within the disparate occupation with hospital nursing, and general hospital nursing in particular, at the apex. The recruitment and selection process outlined in this chapter was only part of a larger process of 'occupational imperialism', and in the next chapter another aspect, the creation of a trained 'elite', will be discussed.

NOTES

1. Dr. Bedford Fenwick, Registration of Nurses, 1905, p. 2.
2. Voysey, Hints, p. 3
3. Evidence of Mr. Malhado, Select Committee on the Metropolitan Hospitals, 1890/1, xiii, p. 125.
4. Such women who would stay on to the end "of a system of discipline and application to duty". Hobbs, Registration of Nurses, 1904, p. 72
5. Evidence of Miss Stansfield, Royal Commission on the Poor Laws, 1909, xxxvii, p. 501.
6. Woodward, To Do The Sick No Harm, pp. 36-8; E. Duncum, 'The Development of Hospital Design and Planning', in Poynter (editor), Evolution of Hospitals, p. 218. Recently, the matron of a large London hospital stated that even now (1979) she was reluctant to recruit locally from what is a depressed, migrant inner city area. (Personal communication).
7. J. Saville, Rural Depopulation in England and Wales 1851 - 1951 (Routledge and Kegan Paul, London, 1957); E. A. Wrigley (editor), Nineteenth-Century Society: Essays in the use of Quantitative Methods for the Study of Social Data (C. U. P., Cambridge, 1972); A. K. Cairncross, 'Internal Migration in Victorian England', Manchester School of Economics and Social Studies, 17, 1949, pp. 67-81.
8. Saville, Rural Depopulation, pp. 31-45.
9. Ibid., pp. 46-7, pp. 88-9, pp. 114-5. See also, J. Cheetham, 'Immigration' in A. H. Halsey (editor), Trends in British Society since 1900 (MacMillan, London, 1972), pp. 468-71. Between 1898 - 1900 the Poplar and Stepney Sick Asylum recruited 66 new probationers: 25 (38%) came from London itself and 6 (9%) from within 50 miles of the capital. Of the rest, 23 (35%) came from over 50 and under 150 miles, and only 3 from Scotland, 1 from Wales and none at all from Ireland. Hospital Records (unpublished).
10. S. A. Tooley, The History of Nursing in the British Empire (Bousfield, London, 1906); H. Morten, How to Become a Nurse (Scientific Press, London, 1895).
11. Dr. Bedford Fenwick, Registration of Nurses, 1905, p.2; Melhado, Metropolitan Hospitals, 1890/1, p. 125; Stansfield, Poor Laws, 1909, p. 501; Abel-Smith, Nursing Profession, p. 47.
12. McBride, Domestic Revolution, Branca, Women; P. Horn, The Rise and Fall of the Victorian Servant (Gill and MacMillan, Dublin, 1975); Ebery and Preston, Domestic Service. For a general discussion of changes in white collar/white blouse work see, L. A. Tilley and J. W. Scott, Women, Work and Family (Holt, Rinehart and Winston, London, 1978), Chapter 7, especially pp. 153-4; pp. 156-162.
13. Mrs. McLellan, 'Oral evidence' (unpublished); Miss

Spyer, 'Oral evidence' (unpublished).

14. Hospital Records (unpublished).

15. Holcombe, Victorian Ladies at Work, Chapter V; Davin, 'Telegraphists', pp. 7-9; M. Bondfield, 'Conditions under which Shop Assistants Work', Economic Journal, June 1899; Fabian Society, Shop Life and It's Reform (1897).

16. Holcombe, Victorian Ladies at Work, pp. 133-6.

17. Partington, Women Teachers, pp. 2-3.

18. The bursary system, introduced in 1907, may have actually inhibited recruitment to elementary teacher training; Partington, Women Teachers, pp. 3-5.

19. Horn, Victorian Servant, p.1.

20. Ebery and Preston, Domestic Service, p. 48.

21. For example - "Miss B. from Windsor; began 2/4/06 - left 16/5/06. Did not wish to train in a Poor Law Institution". Hospital Records.

22. See, for example, Donnison, Midwives.

23. Pinker, Hospital Statistics, p. 57, p. 73, p. 78.

24. Ibid., pp. 61-2, p. 73, p. 75, p. 105; Woodward, To Do The Sick No Harm, pp. 36-7.

25. S. and B. Webb, The State and the Doctor (Longman's, Green, London, 1910), pp. 114-5.

26. Dr. Bedford Fenwick, Registration of Nurses, 1904, p. 12. See also, Evidence of Sidney Holland, Select Committee on Registration of Nurses, 1904, vi, pp. 29-30.

27. Smith, People's Health, pp. 278-284.

28. Burdett, Registration of Nurses, 1905, p. 107; Abel-Smith, Nursing Profession, p. 51.

29. Miss Kenwell, 'Oral evidence' (unpublished).

30. Abel-Smith, Nursing Profession, p. 51.

31. D. Dunkerly, Occupations and Society (Routledge and Kegan Paul, London, 1975), Chapter 1; Stearns, Lives of Labour, pp. 46-7, pp. 59-61.

32. Dunkerly, Occupations, p.5.

33. Hogg, 'Employment', pp. 7-9; Stearns, Lives of Labour, p. 47.

34. McBride, Domestic Revolution, pp. 73-5.

35. Mrs. D., 'Oral evidence' (unpublished); Mrs. Kemp, 'Oral evidence' (unpublished); Mrs. Evenden, 'Oral evidence' (unpublished).

36. Mrs. Maden, 'Oral evidence' (unpublished).

37. E. Ginsberg, Occupational Choice: An Approach to a General Theory (O. U. P., London, 1951).

38. Burdett, Directory, 1898, p. cxxxii, See also, M. Dickens, One Pair of Feet (Penguin, London, 1956) (1980 edition), pp. 8-9; Brook, Nursing.

39. Mrs. Edwards, 'Oral evidence' (unpublished).

40. Mrs. McLellan, 'Oral evidence'.

41. Laurence, Nurse's Life, pp. 1-2. See also, Brook, Nursing, p.1.

42. J. Markham, The Lamp was Dimmed: The Story of a

Nurse's Training (Hale, London, 1975), p. 14.

43. Mrs. Elton, 'Oral evidence' (unpublished).
44. Mrs. Gibbons, 'Oral evidence' (unpublished).
45. Miss Ryder, 'Oral evidence' (unpublished).
46. Abel-Smith, Nursing Profession, p.29.
47. Holland, Registration of Nurses, 1904, p. 57.
48. Burdett, Registration of Nurses, 1905, p. 183.
49. Evidence of Miss Hughes, Select Committee on Registration of Nurses, 1904, vi, p. 80.
50. Evidence of Miss Luckes, Select Committee on Registration of Nurses, 1904, vi, p. 18.
51. Applicant, 'Letter', Nursing Mirror, 6 March 1909, p. 354; A Matron in the West of England, 'Letter', Nursing Mirror and Midwives Journal, 24 January 1914, p. 326.
52. Hospital Records.
53. Evidence of Mr. Rathbone, Select Committee on the Metropolitan Hospitals, 1890/1, xiii, p. 742. Rathbone had been instrumental in persuading Nightingale to 'reform' the nursing at Brownlow Hill Infirmary, Liverpool.
54. Hospital Records.
55. For example: "Kidderminster Union. Probationer Nurses. The Guardians of the above Union require the services of Two Probationer Nurses for the Workhouse, to serve for three years - to take alternate Day and Night Duty - each to receive a salary of £5 p.a. first year; £10 second year; £15 third year, with board (no beer), lodgings, washing and uniform." Poor Law Officers Journal, 10 January 1902, p. 4.
56. For example, S. Hadland, Occupations of Women other than Teaching (Alexander and Shepheard, London, 1886); Dilke, Women's Work; Lady S. Jeune (editor), Ladies at Work (Arnold, London, 1893); M. Bateson (editor), Professional Women upon their Professions (Cox, London, 1895); Phillips, Dictionary; M. M. Bird, Women at Work (Chapman and Hall, London, 1911); E. Morley, Women Workers in Seven Professions (Routledge, London, 1914); E. Adams, Women Professional Workers (MacMillan, London, 1921); Strachey, Careers. See also, H. C. Burdett, The Nursing Profession: How and Where to Train (Scientific Press, London, 1899).
57. Mrs. Maden, 'Oral evidence'.
58. Hospital Records.
59. Mrs. Maden, 'Oral evidence'.
60. Stansfield, Poor Laws, 1909, p. 502.
61. Mrs. W., 'Oral evidence'.
62. Maule, 'Training Schools', p. 70 et seq.
63. Ibid., p. 70 et seq.
64. Hospital Records; Laurence, Nurse's Life, p. 2.
65. Mrs. Hawke, 'Oral evidence'.
66. Hospital Records.
67. Ibid.
68. Ibid.
69. Of course, a high leaving-rate could be financially

useful to the hospital; the non-return of any premium paid
(or only part), no salary during the early months and labour
on the wards at little cost may have prevented some authorities from perceiving a need to reduce these levels. See also,
C. Moore, Skill and the English Working Class 1870 - 1914
(Croom Helm, London, 1980), p. 68.

70. Hospital Records.

Chapter 3

TRAINING AND EDUCATION

> No, I'm not nursing - I'm only doing work I could
> go into service and do.
>
> She cannot escape being turned into a competent
> nurse for the reason that with 30 or 40 beds in a
> ward and only 3 pairs of hands to attend to them,
> she must always be nursing.[1]

Introduction

Broadly speaking, the recruit to nursing between 1881 - 1914
did not conform to the model of an ideal probationer. Individuals may have come close to the stereotype, but many were so
unlike the prescribed type that it is difficult to understand
why they were allowed into the occupation, or why the stereotype survived so intact.

In part the openness of recruitment to general hospital
training came about in response to the increased demand for
nurses in the expanding hospital and non-hospital sectors. As
far as the hospitals were concerned, the need was for the
cheapest form of workforce, women who would work for little
material reward but would also do so for a considerable period
of time.[2] Probationers were therefore taken on for 2, 3 or
even 4 years training, a training which they came to accept in
lieu of adequate wages.

Not all those who began training finished as qualified
nurses; on the way many left the occupation, some for ever. In
the previous chapter we noted the way in which the open door
policy of recruitment was backed up by a selection process
which began with the application form and continued into the
trial period itself. That weeding-out process by which 'unsuitable' candidates were shed served to justify the openness
of nursing: while every woman qua woman might be a nurse to
her family, only those who could develop the skills of the art,
and acquire the knowledge of the science of nursing could be
called professional nurses. This chapter is concerned with
this further stage in the development of the new nurse, and we
shall be looking in some detail at the work of the trainee
nurse, her conditions of employment, and her training programme.

The work of the probationer: the first days

No matter what type of woman slipped through the initial selection process, (or because all types did slip through), the
nurse training period would have to form them into a common

88

mould - to make them general hospital nurses. In that training "metal must be hammered into shape, and human beings must
be subjected to discipline and severe training if they are to
develop the highest type of character or the highest mental
attainments."[3] The woman who passed through such a training
would look back on the experience, "high suffering", and
"thank God" for the way it enabled her to cope with anything
that might happen in her future nursing life.[4]

One way in which we may assess the 'high suffering' of
the probationer is to look at the ratios between nurses and
patients, which might be regarded as indicators of general
changes in nursing levels, although not as descriptions of
standards of nursing care. Table 3.1 gives a superficial account of nurse/patient ratios in our period. Between 1898 and
1905 (data dates) there had been an overall decrease in the
number of patients looked after at any one time by each nurse.
The tendency towards increased off-duty time, more use of more
nurses on night duty, and the expansion of such nursing departments as X-ray and Out-patients, made demands on available
nursing staff which are not reflected in nurse/patient ratios.
These developments influenced the actual nurse/patient contact, that is the length of time each nurse was actually with
a patient. Exaccerbating the problem was the fact that the
number of patients being treated in each hospital increased at
a higher rate than the number of beds provided: shorter pa-
tient-stay acted to reduce the degree of nurse/patient contact.

Caution must be exercised, then, in using such data: indeed, nurse commentators now prefer a new measurement of
nursing practice, the "nurse-hour". In a recent nursing textbook, the authors advised senior nurses to manage their staff
more effectively by costing all nurse activities, including
patient-contact, and to "budget for the expenditure of time",
cut out inefficiency and thus reduce costs.[5] We shall return
to this theme later in the discussion about nursing discipline: here it must be acknowledged that such data only tend
to obscure the widespread experiences of hard work, long hours
on duty and tedious duties which were the lot of contemporary
probationers.

The very first day on duty as a nurse, when the probationer exchanged the "worldly clothes" of the twenty-one year
old woman for the uniform, simple and unadorned, of the novi-
tiate, could be traumatic - so much so that some ran away
rather than face another like it.[6] This semi-fictional account
of one woman's first experiences comes close, however, to the
average for the period:

The wretched little second probationer ragged me
because I did not know the difference between a
'spat' and a 'tongue depressor'. The things I've
learnt in this one week are almost more in number

Table 3.1:   Patient : Nurse [a] Ratios in Selected Hospitals,
             1898 and 1905

Type	Hospital	1898	1905
Voluntary	The London	3.4	2.1
"	Guys	4.6	2.4
"	St. Georges	3.0	2.4
"	St. Mary's	3.8	2.5
"	Newcastle Royal Infirmary	4.5	3.3
"	Birmingham General	4.0	3.4
"	Leicester Royal Infirmary	3.6	3.1
"	Salop Infirmary	5.4	3.8
"	Sussex County Infirmary	3.5	3.1
"	Derby Royal Infirmary	4.7	3.8
"	Bradford Royal Infirmary	4.0	3.8
"	Halifax Royal Infirmary	5.3	4.1
"	Cumberland Infirmary	6.4	4.5
"	Kent and Canterbury Hospital	6.2	4.7
"	Sunderland Infirmary	5.4	4.7
Poor Law	Salford Union	12.5	10.6
"	Whitechapel Union	14.0	13.0
"	Leeds Union	14.0	not avail.
"	St. Marylebone Union	10.3	"
"	Liverpool Workhouse Infirmary	17.7	"
"	Birmingham Poor Law Infirmary	14.7	"

Source: 1898 H. Burdett, Burdett's Official Directory of
          Nurses (Scientific Press, London, 1898).
          1905 Royal Commission of the Poor Law, Vol. LXIV,
          Evidence of Dr. McVail, cited R. White, Social
          Change and the Development of the Nursing Profes-
          sion: A Study of the Poor Law Nursing Services
          1848 - 1948 (Kimpton, London, 1978), pp. 228-29.

   a.   Excluding matrons and assistant matrons.

than the things I find I am expected to know without
learning them ... (The staff nurse) simply sniffed at
me, and said in a cutting tone, "Very well, you can
start the round". I would not ask her what on earth
'the round' meant, but, of course, I had not the fain-
test idea. How that probationer roared when I asked
her! However, whatever else I don't know at the end of
this first week, I know what the 'round' is pretty
thoroughly.[7]

Nurse Hawkins wrote her experiences down for would-be probationers, but if there was any judicious editing, what remained was still a difficult introduction to the work -

My actual work started in a woman's ward. While I was
wondering what I should be expected to do, a nurse
called to me to help her make six of the beds ...
Then followed the dusting of half of the ward, polishing the bedtables and lockers, washing utensils in the
annexes, etc.[8]

Some probationers started on the male wards, which could
be a "bad breaking-in" for those who had led a sheltered life
or had no brothers: others were immediately expected to 'care'
for complex cases, involving the use, for example, of barrier
nursing procedures. Even those with some nursing experience
behind them learnt to keep it hidden during those early weeks,
in particular during the First World War when VADs tried to
move into mainstream nursing.[9] The only women who might not
find the experiences too unnerving were those who paid for
their training, the 'lady pupils' of the voluntary hospitals.
One such, who trained at Guy's Hospital in 1894/5 wrote of
her introduction:

This is a huge place, quite like a little town in
itself and I am very happy here.
    I think I have been lucky in being first sent
to a men's medical ward of 40 beds. The sister is a
first-rate nurse and a splendid manager ... I find
that, as a lady-pupil, I am really acting as 'sister's-
assistant'. I go round with Sister with the doctors
... another of my duties is to give all the medicines
... I also have charge of four beds, and do everything
for the patients in them.
    There are two staff nurses and two probationers
... and I fill in my spare time (sic) with helping them
in bedmaking, carrying round meals etc.; but I don't
seem to be expected to do any of the cleaning work,
and if I am busy helping sister, the routine work goes
on just the same without my assistance.[10]

Being thrown in at the deep end, 'broken in' or helped to find their "sea legs" during those early weeks was not only necessary for the working of the wards - such probationers formed almost the entire 'staff' of most wards[11] - but was another hurdle thrown down in the path of the recruit, another test of 'earnestness'. While some intending probationers had forewarning of the 'trials of the trial period' - "of course, I was warned, and by matron too, at our momentous interview"[12] - the experiences were such that some left before signing their contracts. The high leaving rate, already noted in Chapter 2, points to a rough and rude dissolution of any expectations recruits might have had about nursing, but few contemporary observers considered it to be necessarily bad. Sir Henry Burdett noted that "out of 100 women who applied to be admitted as probationers only 4 became trained and certificated nurses ...", but that this was because many women who wanted to leave home for one reason or another, and who "regard nursing from a distance as an easy and pleasant pastime", found in practice that they were "utterly unsuited" to be trained nurses.[13]

Attempts were made by matrons and hospital authorities to ease the trainee more smoothly into the work, and Preliminary Training Schools, such as the one at The London Hospital (1895), were set up by the voluntary hospitals to reduce the starkness of the contrasts in the initial months of training. Sarah Tooley argued in her study of nursing history that the progress of nurses from the preliminary schools onto the wards was thus made less 'dramatic' -

> no more dummies to bandage and dress, but living patients to deal with now. The work, however, is not so strange as if the probationers had come straight from the parental fireside to the wards. Those 6 weeks ... have taught her what to expect and she enters upon the duties of ward-probationer with a corresponding degree of confidence and facility.[14]

- but such schemes were obviously designed at bringing the entrant to as useful a level as quickly as possible, and not at reducing the high leaving rates.

The work of the probationer: the next three years

There is no lack of evidence about the probationer's life, on- and off-duty, in Poor Law and voluntary hospitals. Many hospitals have produced their own commemorative narrative histories, which usually include at least some anecdotal reference to the nursing staff. Biographical studies often begin with what it meant to do nursing work 'at the bottom', and accounts of probationers' workloads appear in semi- and official reports of contemporary nursing.[15]

Nurse Nettleton began her training when aged 21 years

(1900) at a provincial voluntary hospital: her work, she
recalled, had been "a mixture of helping with patients, scrub-
bing lockers, cleaning brasses, washing tiled walls in sluices
and bathrooms, and emptying bedpans." Treatment of patients
included giving enemata, making poultices, "washing backs, el-
bows and heels and rubbing with methylated spirit and powder,
mornings and evenings."[16]
    Burdett collected information about nursing duties for a
series which appeared in the journal he owned and edited, The
Hospital: the ninth article gave details of the regime at
Guy's Hospital -

> Probationers are called at half-past 6 o'clock in the
> morning, at a quarter-past seven breakfast is served
> in the dining-hall, at a quarter to eight prayers are
> said in the chapel, and at eight o'clock they come on
> duty on the wards. During the morning they clean lamps,
> inkstands, spatulas, etc., thoroughly; dust the ward,
> wash lockers and doctors' tables; wash windowsills;,
> prepare and serve the patients' luncheon; clear lun-
> cheon things; help the nurse with the patients when
> and as required, and assist with the patients' dinner.
> At half-past eleven or at a quarter-past 12 o'clock,
> as arranged by the sister, probationers go to dinner,
> returning to their wards in three-quarters of an hour.[17]

A nurse who trained in a provincial Poor Law Hospital recalled her duties as a probationer -

> every morning the beds were pulled out 12 to 15 inches
> and the nurses swept and dusted at the back of the beds.
> The night nurses were expected to wash and make the beds
> of 8 patients, the day nurses had to do the rest. The
> night nurses gave out the breakfast for 30 patients in
> the ward.[18]

- and she went on to describe in some detail the sort of cleaning she and other probationers had to do each day. However, in
most accounts of wardwork of the period it is possible to dif-
ferentiate between the tasks performed by the different grades
of trainees; there was, that is, a hierarchy of tasks determined by seniority of service and training. "The junior nurse
did many chores", but while the second year nurses also did
"much the same routine", the third year nurses were generally
"busy testing urines, measuring bile or preparing enemata,
douches, colonic washouts and the 101 things" common to any
busy ward.[19]
    A distinction was made also between the work of the day
nurse and that of the night nurse, irrespective of seniority.
All ordinary, i.e. non-paying, probationers were required to do
night-duty, normally alternating 3 months on day-duty with 3

months on nights. Lady pupils, who paid for their training, could opt not to do night-duty, although most matrons were reluctant to give certificates of training to women without such experience.

The night nurses were supervised by either a night sister or night superintendent who visited each ward on her 'round', but the actual work was performed, as during the day, by the nurse-in-training. Night sisters were usually recently qualified nurses awaiting a day sister's post, and hence had little more knowledge or skill than some of the nurses they were supervising. The night nurse, both the probationer and the qualified nurse, was, however, ultimately responsible to the day sister on whose ward she worked - "the night nurse is responsible for carrying out the orders of the day sister under the direction of the night sister".[20]

The work carried out by the night nurses was generally described a 'sandwich' - two brief periods of relatively frenetic activity interspersed by a long middle watch of relative inactivity. It was during this 'filling' time that the greatest challenge to the integrity of the night nurse came:

> when all the patients are asleep ... and during the nurse's rounds of the ward she passes an empty bed, a couch or an armchair ... And now sleep suddenly attacks her with all its force. Nothing seems to rouse her. She is alone in the ward. The quiet breathings of the patients are so many tempting voices. Her eyes ache with weariness. Her eyelids droop, leaden-weighted. She staggers and nearly sleeps as she walks ... she would almost sell her soul to sleep.[21]

The night nurses, as on day-duty, had to remember her earnest desire to become a trained nurse, resist the temptation to end up like Sairey Gamp: she had to be strong in "moral courage", to have the "highest motives". During this testing time the nurse should reject the temptations of the night, and either take the opportunity to "fad over the patients who are really bad and to do little things for their comfort" or to carry out all those cleaning tasks which the day-sister usually required of her night nurses. She should, that is, remember that the 'devil makes work for idle hands.'[22]

For many night nurses the approach of the day nurses was viewed with a mixture of relief and apprehension. It was common practice for there to be an overlap, usually of an hour, when night and day nurses worked together "in the morning when the work is heavy."[23] However, the scrutiny of the night's work by the day sister when she arrived had to be faced by the night nurse alone. The night nurses at Mrs. Richards' hospital were officially off-duty at 8 a.m., but the ward sister "did a round with the night nurse ... and sister checked each patient ... and further comments were entered in the margin of the Night Report." Such a routine meant that the earliest the night nurse could leave the ward was 8.15 a.m., and often it was much later than that.[24]

Hours of duty varied only marginally between hospitals in the period 1881 - 1914. At the Manchester Royal Infirmary (1890) nurses came on duty at 7 a.m. and went off at 9 p.m.: the only change which had taken place by 1914 was that the day ended at 8 p.m.[25] Miss Schofield, who trained at the Westminster Hospital in 1879, worked from 7 a.m. until 8 p.m.; Miss Stollard worked from 6.30 a.m. until 9 p.m. in the Leeds Royal Infirmary around 1912.[26]

The hours between going on duty at 7 a.m. and leaving the ward at 9 p.m. were not spent in continuous ward work: there were meal breaks; time to change uniform or aprons after the heavier cleaning tasks had been finished, and increasingly, periods of off-duty time. By the turn of the century, "a great improvement" had taken place in the provision of off-duty time: "high-water mark is reached with a daily 4 hours off-duty, a half day a week, a whole day once a month and 3 weeks to a month's annual leave."[27] Holcombe has argued that between 1880 - 1914 "nurses' hours were gradually shortened considerably";[28] however, the eight-hour day, a contemporary issue, was not discussed by nurses themselves until 1921 at the earliest;[29] and the available data suggests that while a reduction in the total hours worked by probationers in the voluntary hospitals had taken place, there was an increase in those worked in the Poor Law hospitals. (Table 3.2). In neither sector can we see a significant shortening of the nurse's day and many of the changes which had taken place were probably aimed at lengthening the meal breaks, something which Burdett and others had complained of for years.[30]

However, even when support for a reduction in hours was forthcoming, it was not unequivocal; too much of a reduction was as bad a management practice as having too long a working day, at least according to Burdett.[31] The median was to be arrived at by balancing the physical depredation caused by excessively long hours on duty with the advantages which these contributed to continuous patient care: thus

> it is generally allowed that 10 hours a day in the wards is not too long a time, and that to reduce the hours below this point would have very serious disadvantages, and not be calculated to promote the best interests of either the nurses, the patients or the hospital.[32]

When the nurse, on day or night duty, left the ward at the end of her shift, it was to return to the Nurses' Home. The development of compulsory living-in for probationers, and

Table 3.2: The Average working week of Probationer-nurses in selected hospitals, 1898 and 1908 (hours per week)

Hospital	1898	1908	Reduction
Guys Hospital	87.0	85.0	-2.0
The London	81.0	81.0	nil
Birmingham General	82.25	80.75	-2.5
Royal South Hants	79.5	75.0	-4.5
St. Mary Abbotts (Poor Law)	86.0	86.0	nil
Poplar and Stepney Sick Asylum	80.0	82.0	+2.0
Leeds Union Infirmary	77.25	78.0	+0.75
Sheffield Union Infirmary	78.0	79.5	+1.5

Source: 1898 H. Burdett, Burdett's Official Directory of Nurses (Scientific Press, London, 1898)

1908 L. Maule, 'Training Schools and Other Nursing Institutions' in The Science and Art of Nursing (Cassells, London, 1908), pp. 66-85.

indeed for all grades of hospital nurses, grew out of the
original Nightingale reforms, although the objectives for providing accommodation had undergone considerable adaptation.

In her Training of Nurses (1882) Nightingale had listed
six characteristics which made up a "Good training-School for
Nurses". The sixth characteristic was the provision of "accommodation for sleeping, classes, and meals; arrangements for
time-off and teaching and work; surroundings of a moral and
religious, and hard-working and sober, yet cheerful tone and
atmosphere." Such accommodation would be more than a dormitory,
it would be a "home" whose "motherly influence" would provide
"good women of any class" with a sanctuary from the struggle
against disease.[33]

The Home for the St. Thomas's nurses, funded by the
Nightingale Fund, provided not only sleeping and dining facilities, but also "guided study hours, singing and Bible classes and a sympathetic homelike atmosphere", which went some
way towards allaying the fears of the middle class parent
whose daughter suddenly announced she was going to be a nurse.
[34] But this 'home life' could only be possible if the time
spent in the Home was long enough to allow such activities to
take place; hence, the 60 hour week for probationers at St.
Thomas's from the start of its training. It also implied a
fairly small number of nurses under close supervision, and
while the other hospitals might have been able to provide the
supervision in the form of several Home Sisters - "moral po-
lice"[35] - few could match the funds of St. Thomas's and fewer
still afford to 'waste' it on frivolous pursuits for the probationers.

By the turn of the century, most hospitals had some sort
of Nurses' Home in the Poor Law sector, where £14,350 was
spent in 1900 on a new home for nurses at the Sheffield workhouse, for example.[36] The Western Infirmary, Glasgow, was held
up as a model by Burdett, since it provided "dining rooms and
sitting rooms and class-rooms for the nurses and every nurse
has a separate bedroom to herself."[37]

The Nurses' Home was, like the early Victorian home itself, a haven from work (although in this case, a haven for
the woman and not the man)[38]: Miss Luckes, Matron of the
London Hospital said that the Home provided for the needs of
the nurses, so that "they, being cared for themselves, shall
be ready to devote themselves with all the more energy to the
care of the patient."[39] For most nurses, however, the Nurses'
Homes were another part of the nursing regime of discipline,
where even when nominally off-duty they were still subject to
scrutiny and assessment, where infringements of the rules
could be as significant as mistakes with the patients, and
where privacy was at a premium. It was also the place and the
time when the probationer received her formal instruction in
nursing.

The formal training of the probationer

Leaving the ward at 8 or 9 p.m. the probationer had not finished her long day, even if her physical labours might be over.
It was at that time that the lecture programme was generally
scheduled, each class lasting for at least an hour. Night
nurses were not exempt, and attended lectures in the first
hour after they finished on the wards, or even with the day
nurses on their nights-off. Only those lectures given by the
senior medical staff were held during the day, usually during
one of the off-duty periods, for example, between 2 and 4 p.m.

It was common practice for the larger hospitals, at least,
to print their syllabus(es) of training, which were used in
the many guides to nursing of the time. Reading of lectures in
anatomy, physiology, hygiene and dietetics the potential recruit or her parents could hardly fail but to be impressed by
the depth and breadth of knowledge the 'modern' nurse was expected to acquire. Complex scientific terms were used for what
were often commonplace disorders - haemoptysis for nose bleed
- and even the cleaning tasks took on special significance
when described as part of the nurse's duties as "an active
agent in carrying out 'rest'".[40]

Publication of the syllabus also tended towards standardisation of the formal lecture and instruction programme, since
those hospitals which did not initially detail their training
programme were forced to start to do so when the competition
for recruits developed. Such hospitals often drew on the already published syllabuses, which were those of the larger and
more prestigious voluntary hospitals. While time has obscured
their origins, many hospitals in both voluntary and Poor Law
sector came to offer very similar training programmes, with
some allowance made for local needs and constraints, such as
the availability of medical staff to lecture in the Poor Law
hospitals.[41]

As well as the raw recruit being impressed by the training offered in these printed syllabuses, the nurse thinking of
moving from another area of the occupation to general nursing
could read them and decide whether she could cope with the
training. Since many of these women had not had any formal instruction in their specialist skills, the mere fact that
general nursing was so organised and structured as to offer a
course of instruction and examination may have persuaded some
of the 'superiority' of general hospital nursing.

The movement of staff between hospitals and between voluntary and Poor Law sectors also helped in the promulgation of a
standard training syllabus. This mobility of trained nurses
will be discussed in terms of career patterns in the following
chapter: there is no doubt that when new matrons were appointed
they tended to bring with them the values and methods of their
last post and their own training schools.[42] Where the medical
staff had control over the syllabus, as at the Manchester Royal
Infirmary, the doctors could introduce material they had used

or been familiar with at their training hospitals, i.e. the voluntary hospitals in particular.[43]

Much of the content of nurse training syllabuses came directly from contemporary medical knowledge and practice. Occasionally, the vagaries of medical fashion could invade the nurse training programme, resulting in nurses acquiring knowledge and skills inappropriate to their needs in the occupation as a whole. Thus some hospitals taught their nurses the use of electricity in post-operative and medical conditions, while others taught massage at a time when it was generally acknowledged that it had gone out of fashion, and at a time when the 'trained' masseuse was evolving into the physiotherapist of today.[44]

The nursing content of the training was also informed by medicine, since much of the activity of nursing was geared toward caring for a patient.[45] However, some parts of the syllabus owed more to contemporary domestic science than medicine, even if public health science underpinned domestic science itself. Indeed, the ease with which some nurses apparently became teachers of domestic science subjects, (see below), would tend to confirm the similarities, and many of the nursing textbooks themselves contained much which any reader might find in a manual of home management or in the advice columns of contemporary women's journals.

Some of the earlier textbooks were little more than tracts aimed at improving the general status of the nurse in the public eye;[46] others were upgraded manuals of hygiene for women in general, with an introduction in which the role of the nurse was forcibly argued as being separate from that of the doctor, although both were complimentary in the preservation of life and relief of distress.[47]

Towards the end of the nineteenth-century, nursing textbooks became more elaborate and aimed specifically at the growing army of 'professional' nurses. We lack an analysis of nursing textbooks and their relationship to the occupation, pace Jarman's study which ends in 1895 just when general hospital nursing as a large scale trained occupation was taking off. However, from about 1895 nursing textbooks began to proliferate, and were now written not only by doctors but by trained nurses themselves.

Earlier textbooks had had to rely on doctors' perceptions of what nurses ought to learn and to do: with the introduction of the nurse-author, textbooks still spent some time delineating the respective roles of doctor and nurse, but now included very detailed instructions in nursing procedures, usually those practised by the author in her own hospital.[48] After the turn of the century nursing textbooks rarely referred to Florence Nightingale as the source for the rationale for nursing actions and roles, as those written by Dr. Munro and Dr. Lewis had done. The criteria for judging effectiveness in nursing was no longer simply moral rectitude, but medical science itself.

Hence authors of this new type of book spent long passages on explanations for actions, whether it was the need to open windows at specific times during the day, to properly prepare the skin before an operation, or even to prepare the patient mentally for an operation.[49]

The lectures which made up the larger part of the formal training programme were generally divided by year of training and between those given by the doctors and those by the senior nurses. In the first year the lectures were on basic tasks and skills which the nurse needed in order to do her daily work and included such topics as bedmaking, bandaging, the management and prevention of bedsores, first aid and the application of hot and cold poultices. Most, if not all, of these early lectures were given by nurses; only if they included lectures on anatomy or physiology were the medical staff involved. During the second and third years the nursing lectures continued to stress the application of knowledge through nursing skills, while the medical and surgical lectures were given by the doctors. The distinction was often made in the programme between "practical classes" and "theoretical lectures",[50] the province of the nurse and the doctor respectively. In the Poor Law hospitals, however, such a distinction was not always practical, since there were fewer doctors to give the lectures: the nurses who took such classes were at pains to emphasise the relative spheres of doctor and nurse throughout the course of instruction, and the influence of the medical superintendent over the training of Poor Law nurses was increased by this necessary distancing.[51]

Whenever a lecture was given by a doctor the probationers were chaperoned by the senior nurse responsible for their formal education. These senior nurses were present at each lecture to do more than maintain the proprieties of behaviour: after each doctor's lecture the senior nurse would proceed to either 'review' the content of the lecture or to give a practical class involving the lecture material. This served three important ends: it allowed the probationers to ask questions they might have been afraid to ask the lecturer for fear of appearing dull or out of awe for the medical man; second, it reinforced the distinction between medical and nursing expertise, especially when the lecture was followed by a practical class; and third, it allowed those who had been unable to follow the lecture, which might have been couched in medical terminology, to go over the subject again in more everyday language. While some doctors went to great lengths to enable the probationers to understand medical science, using slides, manikins and dissections to illustrate their topics, others merely rushed in to the room, delivered a barely audible and incomprehensible talk and then ran out before questions could be asked.

Nurses in training were often encouraged to keep notebooks in which they recorded the content of the lectures and practical classes: for the nurses at St. Thomas's these notebooks also had to include details of their wardwork, and this was copied by a few voluntary hospitals as well.[52] More commonly found in the uniform pocket of the trainee was one of the many vade mecum or pocket nursing dictionaries then being published.[53] Such books were very popular, one selling 100,000 copies in eight years and going through several editions, and as such probably played a more important role in nurse training than their authors originally intended.

However the probationer acquired her knowledge, whether it was through the lectures, the practical classes, the textbooks or the aides-memoire in their pockets, the test of the acquisition was the examination system. No training programme ended without a formal examination, usually written and oral, and most were examined at stages throughout the training. As Miss Maule wrote, the period was "an age of examinations, and nursing is no exception to this rule".[54] The granting of a certificate of training could only be justified, according to the general hospital matrons, if it was based upon a programme of instruction and examination -

> Every hospital of repute has examinations for its nurses during their training ... (a) test of technical skill is naturally essential before a certificate of efficiency can be granted. Even given the personal qualities which make a woman a good nurse, if she be unable to give simple proof of having assimilated the instruction given during a course of years, it is clear that she cannot attain the standard which alone can justify an institution to hallmark her as 'trained'.[55]

In a few hospitals an examination was set at the end of the trial period and was one more hurdle that the recruit had to surmount, although the test was usually of general knowledge or simple skills such as cookery. The standard examined in each test reflected the content of the course of lectures or length of training received, and the papers were divided to reflect the different topics covered by the nurse and the doctor instructors. Where no separate questions were set by the nursing staff, an oral examination or practical test was set by the matron. Almost universally the final examination was followed by a viva voce examination conducted either by the doctor alone, or by the doctor and matron together.[56]

Passing the examinations, and in particular the final one, was a pre-requisite to certification. Failure was not unexpected, however, nor necessarily the end of that nurse's training. Re-sits were allowed and only occasionally did they mean an extension to the total length of training. Examiners were able to override the examination results where they thought it necessary to allow a nurse to 'graduate' or to pass on to the

next stage in their training.[57] The pass-rate, as far as it is
possible to assess it, ranged between 78% and 100% (mean average 92%) in the London hospitals and an average of 96% in the
provinces.[58] It would seem that providing the probationer managed to survive the early traumas of training and didn't become one of the leavers, the chances of finishing the training
without a certificate were minimal. Some hospitals overcame
the problem of nurses who were not quite up to first class
standard but who still merited certification by having certificates in classes, first and second: others went so far as to
have classes of training in theory and practice, so that a
nurse might emerge with a first class certificate in theory
and a second class in practice.

The formal education of the probationer, through lectures,
practical classes etc., and tested by examinations, was com-
plemented by the routine performance of nursing tasks on the
wards (see above and below). The training programme, like the
nursing routine, worked to overcome the difficulties experienced by probationers as they moved around the hospital's wards
and departments, to reduce the severe consequences which a
high wastage rate or turnover in personnel might threaten, and
to help newcomers be more easily and quickly familiarised and
assimilated into the hospital and nursing hierarchy.[59]

Informal education of the probationer

The discussion about probationer training in the general hospitals has so far dealt with what contemporaries called the
science of nursing; that is, the rational, medical and biological explanations and justifications for nursing practice.
There existed, however, a complementary system of training,
one which was less clearly formulated but which was nevertheless crucial to the development of modern nursing - the Art of
nursing.

Florence Nightingale had written (1882) that nursing was
an art which required training to fulfil its role as the
"skilled servant of medicine, surgery, and hygiene". Earlier
in the period she had claimed that if it was an art, then it
required "as exclusive a devotion, as hard a preparation, as
any painter's or sculptor's." Nursing proper, that is nursing
the sick and injured as opposed to one's own family as a loving daughter, wife or sister, required skilled practitioners -
hospital trained nurses working under the instruction of doctors.[60]

The born nurse did not exist, according to the authors of
nursing textbooks and nurse reformers like Nightingale: "people may be born with some of the necessary qualities which
make it easy for them to acquire the skill and knowledge ...
to become good nurses"; such natural gifts needed to be drawn
out by proper training, because "nursing, as any other profession, is very much a matter of brains, hard work and common
sense."[61]

102

It is comparatively easy to distinguish what the nurse
did when she was using the science of nursing - taking temperatures, testing specimen, giving out medicines and so on. It is
less certain what she was doing when she was practising her
art; mere performance of nursing tasks - "the mechanical side
of nursing" - was not the art of nursing. The true art, and
the real purpose for nursing, was "the human side of the work",
that is, the personal interactions and relationships in the
world of sickness which formed between the nurse, her nursing
superiors, the doctors and the patients.[62]

In order to perfect the human side of nursing the would-
be nurse had to be, from the first, of "the highest class of
character".[63] In other words, the art of nursing addressed itself to the specific personal qualities of the entrant, rather
than her ability to take in the formal education, although
possession of those qualities would enable her to take best
advantage of the training on offer.

The earliest, and subsequently the definitive, version of
the personal qualities needed were set out in the syllabus of
training of St. Thomas's Hospital for the Nightingale probationers.[64] Those requirements, which included sobriety, honesty, punctuality, truthfulness and patience, were "found
often intact, or more or less embodied in the existing regulations of countless hospitals".[65] However, the Nightingale code
did not emerge in a vacuum, but was adapted from existing
regulations for workers in contemporary prisons and workhouses,
organisations which like nursing had been 'reformed' to stamp
out corruption and malpractice.[66]

To the working matron, as opposed to the public relations
worker, these characteristics were ideals to be striven for or
inculcated into her trainees, rather than descriptions of
actual probationers. Miss Luckes, matron of The London Hospital, wondered

> how many women who entered a hospital with the object
> of acquiring a technical knowledge of nursing, can
> call all these indispensable qualities their own? ...
> everyone will admit that the possession of all of
> them is rather the exception than the rule.[67]

The selection process we have noted would ensure, it was
thought, that only those candidates who had the "fundamental
qualities" of the Nightingale code and a "moderate amount of
intellect and virtue" would become probationers.[68] The hospital life and the work of nursing would draw out those talents
to their fullest extent and at the same time help the girl deficient in any particular quality to acquire it by the culti-
vation of "good nursing habits".[69]

The hospital world was a strict hierarchy of responsibility and duty between doctors and nurses and between trained
and untrained nurses. Any attempts on the part of the trainee

to question or reject that order had to be immediately given up:

> Owing, possibly to the radical tendencies and educa-
> tion of the present day, the virtue of obedience -
> implicit, unquestioning obedience - to superiors is
> somewhat rare and difficult to learn, unless it has
> become a habit from the nursery ... the idea of
> equality is so deeply ingrained, that when we find
> ourselves in an institution where there are neces-
> sarily differences of order, we feel strange, and are
> very much inclined to be rebellious in idea if not in
> act. This must be conquered and that quickly, for no
> learning and no progress will come otherwise. (empha-
> sis added)[70]

To Miss Voysey, writing her textbook for nurses, the good character of the nurse was more important than "all our learn-ing", meaning "book learning": Burdett felt it to be of para-mount importance to a woman following "one of the most noble callings"; nursing was "one of the most purifying and enobling moral disciplines to which a human being can be subjected."[71]
The method by which good nursing habits, i.e. character, were to be produced or encouraged to flower was referred to by contemporaries as hospital etiquette. It was, as one texbook put it, "little more than the ordinary courtesy to which any well-brought-up girl is accustomed in her own home circle".[72] While most nursing guides included a section on good behaviour - standing up in the presence of senior nurses and doctors; never speaking to a senior unless spoken to first, etc. - the code of behaviour to be followed in the individual hospital was never written down. For most probationers the complexity of the code of behaviour only became apparent when it was breached and perhaps a punishment meted out:

> I went to the Matron, to her office. 'Good morning,
> Matron' - and sister would say 'You don't speak to
> Matron, you speak to staff nurse, then staff nurse
> speaks to sister, then sister speaks to Matron.'
> We were not allowed to be friends with the doctors
> or students, it was a crime almost, you were puni-
> shed. For one probationer who went to the Sceptre
> (cinema) with a male student who was a friend of the
> family of long-standing, Matron gave her no off-duty
> for three days as a punishment.[73]

Failure to observe the code could imply high-spiritedness or youthful excess, particularly in the Nurses' home, and as such could be forgiven by the senior nurses who would turn a blind eye to such behaviour which it was felt was almost a natural reaction against the strict tidiness and orderliness required of the nurse on the ward.[74]

But failure to maintain the hospital discipline and etiquette could also imply a failure of moral character. A nurse who sinned might be able to pass an examination in technical knowledge but she could never be a "true nurse" only a "mechanical nurse" -

> Mechanical nurses can be produced by machinery. But what kind of a substitute is a human machine for a tender-hearted woman, who, from practical training and experience, is skilled in the services and attention which sick people require, and whose devotion to her work is inspired by a genuine love of, and satisfaction in helping, those who are in need of what she has to give?[75]

The code of behaviour was unwritten and could only be learnt by making mistakes; the probationer who did not fall foul of the system must therefore be a "true nurse" with a good character, although how many were such paragons is difficult to estimate. There was another way in which the new probationers could develop their moral characters, and that was through the acceptance and application of a time-orientated existence, on- and off-duty. The importance of time in nursing practice cannot be over-stated;[76] it was the use of time which contributed towards the production of a standard hospital nurse through the routine of ward work and even off-duty life. As one nurse recalled, she had liked nursing because "you knew the hours, and I liked the routine very much."[77]

At one level the use of time, by the trained nurse in particular, served to produce order out of chaos: according to one doctor

> the importance of the nurse recalls Darwin's observation of a slave-ant, introduced into a company of helpless starving master-ants, instantly set to work, fed and saved the survivors, and put all to rights.[78]

- and a recent author (1964) claimed that the Nightingale reforms had meant that "nursing duties were carried out at a smarter pace, slovenly techniques had been replaced by rigid rituals."[79]

As we have seen in the discussion of probationers' duties, time provided the framework for the tasks of the nurse at all levels of responsibility. It also ordered the patients' day, which was well-regulated albeit punctuated by long periods - "interminable hours" - of boredom and inactivity.[80] In-patients had only the activities of others to tell them what time it was; the most obvious of those activities being associated with waking-up; mealtimes; ablutions and elimination;

treatments and visits by the doctors. The timing of these
events was determined less by the needs of the patient and
more by the time-orientated routines of nursing tasks. As one
ex-patient recalled, "it still seemed strange to me not to be
washed at 4 a.m. and fed at 6 a.m." when she returned home.[81]
    The importance of time and its impact on nursing practice
and hence nurse training was emphasised throughout contemporary nursing literature. It appeared as a virtue to be cultivated or as something which had been wasted, lost or which had
somehow passed too quickly before everything had been completed. The secret of good ward management, according to Doctor
Lewis, was order and punctuality -

> Meals and medicines, changes of poultices and fomen-
> tations, dressings, washings, dusting, everything
> that takes place in a ward, should have a fixed time,
> and should be done to the minute. (original emphasis). [82]

    - and Miss Fox, a nurse writer of textbooks, advised the
probationer to "try to get your work done to time, so that you
are ready at the proper minute." Even the most mundane tasks,
such as giving out bedpans and urinals, had to be 'done to
time': indeed, most hospitals had "fixed hours ... appointed
for this work" which had to be adhered to for the sake of
"general order and convenience (sic) of all".[83]
    Adherence to a systematic order and routine of work -
even to the extent of having fixed times when the patients'
bladders were expected to function - served not only the needs
of the hospital and the ward, but provided the future trained
general hospital nurse with a degree of superiority if she left
the hospital for private nursing. The method she had learnt in
her work during her training would enable her to perform her
duties with the least labour and in the shortest time, 'skills' which would endear her to her cost-conscious employers.[84]
    Under the old system of nursing time passed by the nurses,
especially since under that system the nurse had merely watched
the struggle between life and death, health and disease. The
new system, with the transformation of mere watching into scientific observation and intervention, turned the nurse into an
active worker, a user of time. Some aspects of this scientific
observation were carried out as 'rounds', often processional
events which ritually took up time in their performance. Increasingly, such events came to be made up of tasks delegated
or relegated by the doctors to the nurses, including the taking of temperatures or the giving of medicines.[85] The original
observations which Nightingale had stressed as being the real
province of the nurse - the minutiae of observations of the
colour of the skin, condition of the nails, mouth, breath etc.
- were not given the time to be specific 'rounds'. Such observations had therefore to become part of the nature of the
nurse, performed unconsciously while she was doing something

else: until they were second-nature junior probationers were urged to "use your eyes and other senses. Keep your minds fixed on what you are doing when at work ... Carry on your observations all the time you are washing ... a patient", for example.[86]

Despite a plethora of advice, nurses on the wards continually "ran out of time": even the nurse who might try to anticipate a little could not get it right

> You used to go on to a ward and the sister would say 'What time are you on duty, nurse?', and you used to say 'Seven o'clock, sister.' 'It's two minutes to seven; go outside and come in at the correct time'. You had to be completely on the dot.[87]

Punctuality was an aspect of the twin virtues of order and method which informed not only observation but all nursing activities, including getting up in the Nurses' Home: failure to be puntual was punished - "we were called at 6 o'clock and went down to breakfast at 6.30 a.m. We had to sign a book and if we were late three times in one week we forfeited one half-day".[88] Nurses, probationers and even qualified nurses, "lived by the clock" and "time had to be kept to the minute".[89]

The new system of nursing transformed time itself into a commodity whilst continuing to call it a virtue; it could therefore be claimed that the good nurse, the efficient new nurse, utilised her time well. While never cutting corners she was always able to keep up with the clock, up to time. The inefficient, bad nurse always ran out of time; however, the junior nurses also complained of not having enough time or of time flying past them. For these nurses the explanation was offered that they were indeed junior and had not yet cultivated the good habits of the trained nurse; if they wished to become good nurses they should learn to use time well.[90]

If a junior probationer rejected such advice she faced reprimand and punishment, even if she felt she did so for 'humanitarian' reasons - " ... there was a recognised time to give out the bedpans. But if a patient called out and said, 'Nurse, could I have a drink of water?' or 'Nurse, could I have a bedpan?', I used to go and take it to them. I got into no end of trouble serving between times."[91]

To stop working and talk to a patient was not allowed even if the nurse had 'time' to do so. Time spent in talking to the patients could be considered by senior nurses as time lost or wasted, literally mis-spent. In part this was because the nurse was now an active agent expected to be on the go all of the time; it was also because talking to patients had connotations of familiarity and flirtation - "you hardly dared stop and talk to a patient, you know, or you'd be accused of getting familiar with them".[92] Enid Bagnold had found such an attitude when she was a V.A.D. nurse during the First World War,[93] as have all subsequent generations of nurses, much to the delight and profit of writers of fiction.

The ward routine, determined by the clock and the hospital etiquette, worked to produce order and method in an environment which was not in itself ordered. Few patients arrived on a planned basis, most being admitted either as accidents, emergencies or through out-patient clinics. The course of each illness, even when controlled to a degree by drugs or operative measures, was largely unpredictable and the patients highly individualistic sufferers despite the hospital routine. At the apex of that control and utilisation of time was the ward sister, the nurse who seemed to be above time, often literally in the sense that her office was beyond the ward doors and the ward clock over them. She had no time-consuming routines to perform, the junior nurses and the staff nurse did those: she even came on to the ward after the heavier work of the nurses was completed by the juniors. The ward sister could stand or sit apart from the melee, superintending, managing, creating order through her orders, even to the extent of enshrining those orders into her own ward routine, rather than daily repetition of specific instructions.[94] The ward sister regulated the work of the ward by timetabling tasks which, as we have noted, ensured their completion: meals were given out; backs washed and rubbed; bedpans and urinals given out and collected, all to time. By thus breaking up the day into routine activity the ward sister and the hospital authorities themselves were able to manage the hospital effectively. One of the major criticisms levelled at the old-style nurses had been that "they had no fixed hours of work ..., they came into the wards when they pleased and practically they went out when they pleased": no hospital administrator could allow such extravagence under the new cost-conscious order. Time was money and the nurses had to spend it wisely.[95]

Conclusion
The occupation itself came to admit that despite an initial influx of a few middle-class women, the profession of general hospital nurse was "mixed as to rank".[96] Whatever the social origins of the recruit, however, the matrons were sure that they could improve "inferior material" by "instilling a high tone and ideals" during the training years. Where the fault lay in the lack of home training - "few girls were taught to respect and obey their parents", lamented one matron - order and courtesy could be inculcated through training in etiquette.[97]

In order for such "weak raw material" to be turned into trained nurses hurdles had to be placed in their paths;[98] some of the very weakest had to fail in order to justify the success of the survivors and legitimate the harsh training regime. Such hurdles included the selection process and the trial period, which we have discussed; some women failed, however, because they were unable to pass the ultimate test of the new order of nursing, the need to work at a very smart pace; for example -

> Dismissed for being hopeless, unpunctual and careless. Dismissed. Good to patients, does not keep up to time. Very dissatisfied with herself. This probationer suffers from her early home training. She is totally ignorant of the most simple household duty. She is willing to be taught <u>but there is no time to teach her to do this</u>. Her nursing has, therefore, suffered. Dismissed. (emphasis added).[99]

The probationer who survived the trial period and the training itself was likely to be the woman who had enough "commonsense to learn from her fellow-nurses the routine of the ward and (to) quickly fall in line". She was in consequence the woman who despite being "niggled" by the etiquette which pervaded all activities, liked the way in which "everything went by clockwork". Life for her might have been hard but "the strict routine gave (her) a certain security".[100]

The hospital discipline containing a hierarchy of duties and personnel worked with the formal training programme to justify even the menial jobs of cleaning and polishing, and transform them into the art and science of nursing. The reward held out to the woman involved in this process was the status of a certificated general hospital nurse. Whether that status was worth the long years of training could only be judged by what happened to the certificated nurse after she qualified.

NOTES

1. Mrs. O'Keefe, 'Oral evidence' (unpublished); 'Truth', p. 361.
2. White, <u>Social Change</u>, p. 209; Carter, <u>New Deal</u>, p. 148; Balme, <u>A Criticism</u>, p. 39.
3. Miss Mollett, 'What is the present position of the Nurse in the estimation of the General Public?', <u>British Journal of Nursing</u>, 18 October 1913, p. 311. See also, J. Dewar, 'The Evolution of Nurses', <u>Nursing World and Hospital Review</u>, October 1895, p. 3; A. I. Twitchell, 'The Discipline of the Nurse', <u>American Journal of Nursing</u>, March 1903, pp. 450-54; Meg, 'Four Letters from a Hospital', <u>Nursing Times</u>, 20 April 1907, p. 339.
4. Mollett, 'General Public', p. 311.
5. R. Hoy and J. Robbins, <u>The Profession of Nursing</u> (McGraw-Hill, London, 1979), p. 111.
6. <u>Hospital Records</u>.
7. Meg, 'Letters', p. 317.
8. M. Heather-Biggs, 'The Work of a Hospital Probationer' in <u>Science and Art of Nursing</u>, pp. 125-6. See also, Dickens,

Feet, pp. 24-6

    9. Wilson, Gone with the Raj, p. 6; Laurence, Nurse's Life, p. 63, refers to her previous nursing experience as "having been out before".

    10. Laurence, Nurse's Life, pp. 62-3.

    11. See Chapter 4 for a discussion of staffing levels.

    12. Meg, 'Letters', p. 314.

    13. Evidence of Sir H. C. Burdett, Select Committee on the Metropolitan Hospitals, 1890/1, xiii, Appendix P, pp. 809-13.

    14. Tooley, British Empire, p. 161.

    15. For example, Brockbank, M.R.I.; S. T. Anning, The General Infirmary at Leeds (Livingstone, London, 1963); Wilson, Gone with the Raj; Laurence, Nurse's Life; E. McManus, Matron of Guy's (Melrose, London, 1956); Voysey, Hints; Vivian, Lectures; Evidence of Sir H. C. Burdett, 'Nurses' Work', Royal Commission on the Poor Laws, 1909, xl.

    16. Nettleton, 'Nurses's Life', p. 1615. See also, M. H., 'A Dream', British Journal of Nursing, 3 April 1909, pp. 267-8.

    17. H. C. Burdett, 'The Department of Modern Nursing', The Hospital, 27 February 1915, p. 496.

    18. Miss Ryder, 'Oral evidence'.

    19. Mrs. W., 'Oral evidence'.

    20. Vivian, Lectures, p. 56.

    21. H. Wilson and R. Wilson, 'Hospital Nursing' in Jeune, Ladies at Work, p. 99. See also, Voysey, Hints, p. 100; Vivian, Lectures, p. 57.

    22. Laurence, Nurse's Life, p. 76; Vivian, Lectures, pp. 57-9; Voysey, Hints, pp. 100-102. The theme of 'night' recurs in many warnings given to probationers, through their training and through popular fiction. Night-duty was seen as the period of least nursing activity which enhanced the air of mystery and sexuality of the nurse. It was the time when men and women's social defences against overt sexuality were thought to be at their lowest. See, for example, the novels about nurses set in hospitals at night, including J. J. Abraham, The Night Nurse (Chapman and Hall, London, 1913) (1916 edition).

    23. S.B. Gadgil, 'The Working of an 8-hour day', Nursing Mirror and Midwives Journal, 19 February 1921, p. 272; Vivian, Hints, p. 59. See also E. Meadows, 'A Day in my Life: A Ward Sister's day', Nursing Times, 7 April 1928, p. 405.

    24. Mrs. Richards, 'Oral evidence' (unpublished).

    25. Brockbank, M. R. I., p. 63, p. 103; Nettleton, 'Nurse's Life', p. 1615; Wilson, Gone with the Raj, p. 10.

    26. Schofield, 'Summer's Day', pp. 30-1; Stollard, 'Nursing', np.

    27. Maule, 'Training Schools', p. 56.

    28. Holcombe, Victorian Ladies at Work, p. 79.

    29. Gadgil, '8-hour day', p. 372; Holcombe, Victorian Ladies at Work, pp. 78-80. However, see Third Report, Select

Committee on the Metropolitan Hospitals, 1892, xiii, p. ixxxvi, p. ciii; also, L. Dock, 'The Present Status of the Nurse in the Nursing World', British Journal of Nursing, 3 January 1914, pp. 4-6; Balme, A Criticism, p. 30; Baly, Nursing and Social Change, pp. 233-4; Abel-Smith, Nursing Profession, pp. 55-6.

30. Burdett, Poor Laws, 1909, p. 812.

31. Ibid., p. 812.

32. Ibid., p. 812. See also, Nettleton, 'Nurse's Life', p. 1615.

33. Nightingale, 'Training of Nurses', p. 232.

34. E. R. Barritt, 'Florence Nightingale's Values and Modern Nursing Education', Nursing Forum, 1, 1973, p. 31.

35. For a discussion of this theme see, M. Dean and G. Bolton, 'The Administration of Poverty and the Development of Nursing Practice in Nineteenth-Century England' in Davies (editor), Rewriting, pp. 88-90; C.Davies, 'A Constant Casualty: Nurse Education in Britain and the U.S.A. to 1939' in Davies (Editor), Rewriting, p. 104.

36. Local Government Board, Annual Report, 1884/5, xxxii, p. xxix; Evidence of Mr. Bagenal, Royal Commission on the Poor Laws, 1909, xl, Appendix XV (H), p. 325.

37. Cited in I. Hampton (editor), Nursing of the Sick (McGraw-Hill, London, 1893) (1949 reprint), pp. 141-2.

38. For a discussion of this role see, A. S. Wohl, 'Introduction' in A. S. Wohl (editor), The Victorian Family: Structure and Stresses (Croom Helm, London, 1978), pp. 9-10.

39. Hampton, Nursing, pp. 201-4. This was precisely the role ascribed to the ideal Victorian middle-class wife: freed from the daily grind by servants, she could provide her husband with all his needs and so prevent him going outside of the home and family. See P. Branca, 'Image and Reality: The Myth of the Idle Victorian Woman' in M. Hartman and L. W. Banner (editors), Clio's Consciousness Raised (Harper, New York, 1974), pp. 179-89.

40. Maule, 'Training Schools', pp. 59-60.

41. Stansfield, Poor Laws, 1909, p. 515 et seq.; White, Social Change, pp. 140-1.

42. This was the case at the Royal South Hants. Infirmary, Southampton, where Miss Mollett, Matron (1898), introduced a 3 year training programme.

43. Brockbank, M. R. I., p. 77. The appointment of doctors as external examiners for nurses' examinations is also discussed by Maule, 'Training Schools', p. 61.

44. H. C. Burdett, 'The Department of Modern Nursing', The Hospital, 13 June 1914, p. 301; Maule, 'Training Schools', p. 92; Tooley, British Empire, pp. 334-7; A.Hughes, 'Nursing as a Vocation' in Science and Art of Nursing, p. 108; Matron, How, p. 115.

45. Brockbank, M. R. I., p. 77.

46. No complete study of nursing textbooks exists: for

an analysis of the early manuals see, F. Jarman, 'The Development of Conceptions of Nursing Professionalism among General
Hospital Nurses 1860 - 1895', unpublished MA. thesis, University of Warwick, 1980, Chapter 3. See also, M. Chayer, 'The
Trail of the Nursing Textbook', American Journal of Nursing,
October 1950, pp. 606-7; L. Parr, 'Early Libraries for Nurses
1860 - 1914', Journal of Librarianship, 12, (2), April 1980,
pp. 102-114.

47. For example, A. Munro, The Science and Art of Nursing the Sick (Maclehouse, Glasgow, 1873), "A nurse, or the
woman in charge of the sick, has a somewhat similar relation
to the doctor that the first mate of a ship has to the captain:
each has a proper sphere and duty to do, and neither can be
dispensed with", p. 4. See also, P. Lewis, Theory and Practice
of Nursing (Scientific Press, London, 1893), p. 1.

48. For example, Voysey, Hints; Vivian, Lectures; E. M.
Fox, First Lines in Nursing (Scientific Press, London, 1914);
A. Goodrich, The Social and Ethical Significance of Nursing
(Scientific Press, London, 1914). For a criticism of this type
of manual see, Review of Young, Outlines, in The Hospital, 8
August 1914, p. 533.

49. For example, J. K. Watson, A Handbook for Nurses
(Scientific Press, London, 1899), p. 73, p. 182.

50. Stansfield, Poor Laws, 1909, p. 517.

51. Ibid., p. 517 et seq.

52. Williams, 'Nursing Systems', pp. 70-1.

53. For example, H. Morten, The Nurse's Dictionary
(Scientific Press, London, 1893); E. M. Clarke, The Nurse's
'Enquire Within' (Scientific Press, London, 1906).

54. Maule, 'Training Schools', p. 60.

55. Ibid., pp. 60-1.

56. Tooley, British Empire, pp. 160-161; Stansfield,
Poor Laws, 1909, pp. 516-9; Maule, 'Training Schools', pp. 60-
3.

57. Stansfield, Poor Laws, 1909, p. 526.

58. Ibid., p. 515 et seq. See also, Brockbank, M. R. I.,
p. 98.

59. Burdett, Hospitals and the State, p. 9; Burdett,
'Nurses Food', p. 813; Luckes, Registration of Nurses, 1904,
pp. 170-2; C.Davies, 'Experiences of Dependency and Control in
Work', Journal of Advanced Nursing, 1, 1976, pp. 279-80;
Vivian, Lectures, p. 19.

60. Nightingale, 'Training of Nurses', p. 237; Nightingale, Notes on Nursing, Preface, np. See also, Holcombe, Victorian Ladies at Work, p. 75; P. Bright, The Nurse and Her
World: A Young Person's Guide (Gollancz, London, 1961), p. 32.

61. Lewis, Theory, p. 1; E. Luckes, General Nursing
(Kegan Paul, Trench and Trubner, London, 1898), pp. 3-4;
Hughes, 'Vocation', p. 95.

62. Luckes, General Nursing, p. ix.

63. Nightingale, 'Training Schools', p. 57.

64. Maule, 'Training Schools', p. 57.

65. Ibid., p. 57.

66. An interesting comparison may be made between these regulations and those for the emerging prison officer. Citing G. O. Paul, An Address to His Majesty's Justices of the Peace (1809) and G. O. Paul, Considerations on the Defects of Prisons (1784), Ignatieff argues "Paul was frustrated not only by the resistance of prisoners, but also by the inefficiency of the custodial staff. He had hoped to replace the 'unregulated discretion' of the old keepers with 'mild government by rule' ... (Paul said) 'It was a principal desideration of our undertaking to make a change in the 'race' or kind of man usually chosen for a gaoler or a keeper of a prison, with whose name and office ideas of cruelty and tyranny and oppression were so associated that it was one of the least difficult parts of the undertaking to convince mankind that it was not a necessary association ... The humanity of the gaoler should rather be the result of coldness of character than the effect of a quick sensibility ... he should be endowed with a patience which obstinacy the most pertinacious could not overcome; a sense of order which is method, rather mechanical than reflective and which few men obtain but by long habits of subordination and obedience." M. Ignatieff, A Just Measure of Pain: The Penitentiary in the Industrial Revolution 1750 - 1850. (MacMillan, London, 1978), pp. 103-4.

67. Luckes, General Nursing, pp. 11-12.

68. E. Luckes, What Will Trained Nurses Gain By Joining The British Nurses Association? (Churchill, London, 1889), p. 6.

69. Ibid., p. 6.

70. Voysey, Hints, pp. 5-6; Dickens, Feet, p. 36.

71. Voysey, Hints, p. 8; Sir H. C. Burdett, How to Succeed as a Trained Nurse (Scientific Press, London, 1913), p. 8; Fox, First Lines, p. 3.

72. Vivian, Lectures, p. 26; Voysey, Hints, p. 7: Dickens, Feet, p. 33.

73. Mrs. Davies, 'Oral evidence'; Mrs. Kenwell, 'Oral evidence'. Some early nurses did have a written code: see, Woodward, To Do The Sick No Harm, pp. 30-1.

74. Vivian, Lectures, p. 42.

75. Luckes, General Nursing, p. x. See also, Voysey, Hints, p. 7. The industrial metaphor is continued in the definition of etiquette as "The oil that oileth rusty wheels", Meg, 'Letters', p. 392. See also, Balme, A Criticism, p. 14; Meadows, 'Ward Sister's Day', p. 405.

76. Davies, 'Control', pp. 135-6. The following discussion owes much to E. P. Thompson, 'Time, Work, Discipline and Industrial Capitalism', Past and Present, 38, 1967, pp. 56-97 and S. Pollard, The Genesis of Modern Management: A Study of the Industrial Revolution in Great Britain (Arnold, London, 1965) (1968 edition), Chapter 5.

77. Miss Davies, 'Oral evidence'. See also, V. Brittain, Testament of Youth (Gollancz, London, 1933), p. 209.
78. W. C. Davidson, 'Nursing as the Foundation of Medicine', Trained Nurse and Hospital Review, October 1943, p. 259.
79. Simpson, 'Influence of Professional Nursing', p. 245.
80. H., 'Through the patients' eyes', Nursing Times, 18 June 1921, p. 685.
81. H., 'Patients'', p. 685. See also, B. Aronovitch, Give it Time (Deutsch, London, 1974), p. 42; Vaizey, Institutional Life; Hake, Suffering London, p. 50; Fox, First Lines, p. 23. When asked if the nurses at Guy's Hospital began attending to the patients before 7.30 a.m., Mr. Lushington, Honorary Secretary, replied "Yes; people of the working-classes have been all their lives in the habit of waking very early." Evidence of Mr. Lushington, Select Committee on the Metropolitan Hospitals, 1890/1, xiii, p. 8. See also, Hardy, Yes, Matron, p. 18.
82. Lewis, Theory, p. 4.
83. Fox, First Lines, p. 24, p. 77; 'How to prepare for becoming a Probationer', Nursing Mirror, 7 September 1907, p. 347; Dickens, Feet, p. 32.
84. Watson, Handbook, p. 70.
85. Dr. Bedford Fenwick, Registration of Nurses, 1904, pp. 3-4.
86. Fox, First Lines, p. 72.
87. Mrs. Maden, 'Oral evidence'. See Watson, Handbook, p. 61 for the 'correct' practice.
88. Mrs. Hitchin, 'Oral evidence' (unpublished).
89. Mrs. Hawke, 'Oral evidence' (unpublished); Mrs. Richards, 'Oral evidence'.
90. C. Maggs, 'Control mechanisms and the 'new nurses' 1881 - 1914', Nursing Times, 2 September 1981, p. 99; Fox, First Lines, p. 72.
91. Mrs. Kemp, 'Oral evidence' (unpublished). See also, Brockbank, M. R. I., p. 63.
92. Mrs. Gibbons, 'Oral evidence'.
93. E. Bagnold, Diary Without Dates (Heinemann, London, 1918) (1978 edition), pp. 70-1; Brittain, Testament of Youth, p. 212.
94. Maggs, 'Control mechanisms', p. 99; Carpenter, 'Managerialism and Professionalism', pp. 166-9.
95. Lushington, Metropolitan Hospitals, 1890/1, p. 3; Burdett, Poor Laws, 1909, p. 1; E. Goffman, Asylums: Essays on the Social Situation of Mental Patients and Other Inmates (Doubleday, New York, 1961) (1980 edition), pp. 66-7.
96. Voysey, Hints, p. 3.
97. 'Matrons' Council', British Journal of Nursing, 25 October 1913, p. 334.
98. Ibid., p. 334.
99. Hospital Records.
100. Vivian, Lectures, p. 19.

Chapter 4

CAREERS IN NURSING

> Clad in the garb which, like the academic gown,
> wipes out all social distinction, emphasising only
> scholastic attainments she can go forth to render
> a complete service, the service of mind and heart
> and hand for the physical and social betterment of
> mankind.[1]

Introduction

'Once a nurse, always a nurse' would appear to have been an
important attitude amongst those who sought to make nursing
exclusively a trained occupation. Nursing was like learning
to read - once the elementary skill was acquired through correct teaching it could not be unlearnt or denied, only enhanced through use.

> I should have thought that it was almost impossible
> for a woman who had been thoroughly trained really
> to forget what she had learnt ... I do not think you
> lose a thing that you once thoroughly learnt.[2]

While a refresher course could keep the nurse up to date,
as could her work alongside a good doctor, as long as her
original training had been securely learnt and she had not
spent her life on a "desert island", the trained nurse of the
new order would always be a professional.[3] Even if the nurse
gave up her work to get married, her training went with her,
since it had been part of that training to turn her into a
'good and true woman': contemporaries recommended nurse training for schoolgirls to make them "better" wives and mothers,[4]
and even recent writers echo such sentiments -

> Training as a nurse, even if incomplete, has some
> value as a preparation for motherhood, and the pro-
> fession might be as well to draw attention to this
> aspect of it as to imply that it is a preparation
> for a life-long career. Nurse training is also a
> preparation for citizenship received by about one
> girl in twenty. She can gain from it something analo-
> gous to what young men gain from national service ...
> It is not necessarily wasteful for so many families
> to have a mother or aunt equipped with some knowledge
> of nursing.[5]

Few women appear to have entered nurse training with any clear career in mind, even those making a 'mature choice'. It was the often abrupt end to training, the final examinations, certification and the distinct probability that the hospital would no longer want to employ them that forced most nurses to consider their future, perhaps for the first time in their lives. General hospital trained nurses had at least a certificate of competence which could help them in the world of nursing work; how that training gave them the edge over other 'nurses' forms the subject of this chapter.

Registers and Registration

The issue of the registration of nurses by the State and the political developments which led up to it have rightly been emphasised by those concerned with professionalisation and professional strategies. If nursing established a Register of trained nurses, backed by statute, the occupation could claim exclusive right to provide specific services; exclude those who failed to meet with occupational approval either through lack of training or lack of morals; and control the admission, education and training of future members of the profession.

Nursing shared common strategies for professionalisation with other Victorian and Edwardian groups, including medicine, midwifery, dentistry, teaching and accountancy.[6] Nursing was to a certain extent unique in that it was an almost entirely female occupation, at a time when female occupations were not considered to meet criteria for professional status. This in itself was not necessarily an obstacle in the path of registration strategy; one group excluded when State Registration was introduced (1919) were the male nurses even if they were 'trained', and some recent commentators have adopted the term "semi-profession" to classify such groups as nurses and teachers in the modern period.[7]

State Registration of nurses came about only after a protracted campaign, sectional, bitter and divisive.[8] There were, however, registers of nurses in existence before 1921 when the General Nursing Council first published its statutory list, which despite their limitations did set out to fulfil some of the functions of the later official Registers.[9] They provide the historian, therefore, with a source for a study of occupational mobility, career patterns and, in our case, 'occupational imperialism'.

The first of these registers in England was proposed by Sir Henry Burdett under the auspices of The Hospitals Association in 1887. This proposal met with the qualified support of the Nightingale-faction within the London voluntary hospitals, because it set out to provide only an information bank about 'trained' nurses and did not require some form of examination of competence for inclusion on the register. The register was to be made available to any matron or private individual who might want to hire a nurse; it would list the previous employment of the nurse and include hospital experience where this was appropriate.[10]

The openness of this register, which failed to test the 'suitability' of nurses for inclusion and exclude the 'unfit', made it ripe for attack by those reformers agitating for State regulation of nurses, centred around Mrs. and Dr. Bedford Fenwick, who saw it merely as a "central registry office similar to that in vogue for domestic servants". The pro-Registration faction broke away from Burdett and set up the British Nurses Association, (B.N.A.) which produced its own register. The B.N.A. claimed to be "a union of nurses for professional objects" and sought to exclude from membership as many nurses as it considered unsuitable. After an initial period of grace which allowed one-year trained nurses to register, future 'registered nurses' had to have evidence of at least a three-year training in a 'recognised' hospital and the personal recommendation of a matron as to the nurse's moral character.[11]

Neither register enjoyed much success, although both were published annually: Burdett claimed, for example, that many of the 4,000 names on the B.N.A. register were duplicated on his, and Sidney Holland felt that no-one could ever "make the nurses register compulsorily" if they wouldn't do so voluntarily. In 1905 the Burdett register had 8,000 names, but even Burdett was candid enough to admit that it ought to have "had all the 25,000 or 30,000" trained nurses then in existence on it.[12]

Even when State Registration came into force (1921) resistance to enrolment was commonplace, and many nurses did not even concern themselves about the method of becoming registered, content to leave it to the matron or hospital authorities to ensure their inclusion. Disinterest and open hostility to State Registration extended to the matrons, and had catastrophic results for some nurses trained under such opponents to State intervention. The matron of The London Hospital in the post-First World War period was against registration; as a consequence one State examiner remembered that when "examining in London I came across some quite elderly female nurses, they were at The London, say, and the matron didn't approve of State Registration and they were told there was no need to take the State examinations 'cause it wasn't necessary - they were at a good hospital, a good training school.' Well, they found they couldn't get a good post because they were not State Registered, and then these girls decided later on to take the State examination when they were much older. I have examined several of these and they were very sad about it (sic)."[13]

However, as the Fenwicks had pointed out, registers were very much in fashion among all sorts of workers in the period, and the willingness by even a few nurses to pay an annual fee and to take the trouble to annually re-register suggests that such registers did serve some purpose for contemporary nurses. As well as these 'national' registers there were also the

registers produced by the individual hospital, and these were
probably more effective because they had limited aims. Such
registers listed nurses trained in the hospital, and since
they were not published could also record opinions on the
woman's nursing and moral character which the matron could
refer to later when considering promotion or providing a
reference. In a few hospitals the subsequent career of the
nurse was recorded, and this together with any other publish-
able material relating to the nurse could be reproduced in an
annual newsletter to the 'alumni'.

Registers maintained by the hospitals and the voluntary
associations which were published and circulated served a more
important function than their role in the debate over State
Registration or in acting as employment registers. They served
to show to the nurses themselves the beginnings of a corporate
identity, however fragile it might have been in the midst of
this political battle. Nurses could keep in contact with each
other merely by looking at the latest edition of The Hospital
Letter, Burdett's Directory or The Annual Report of the B.N.A.
They were thus able to follow the careers of women they had
known or trained with and could see themselves perhaps in
similar posts in the world of nursing.

Listing the various employments taken up by 'graduates'
at home and abroad, the registers demonstrated the advantages
which general training offered them and which made the years
of training seem worthwhile. The alma mater served to bind
the occupation together, even if it tended to emphasise individual hospitals rather than national cohesion. This esprit
had already been of value to the doctors,[14] now nurses themselves were urged to develop the 'school-system' since "the
closer the alliance between the nurse and her training school,
the better it is for her welfare, and that of the patients,
and for the general good of the profession and the public".[15]

The registers, the Nurses Leagues which grew out of the
training school system and the associations for professional
purposes, helped to fill a gap which existed between many
nurses' expectations and the realisations of the use-value of
probationer training. They allowed the newly-trained nurse to
see why she had through the "high suffering" of training and
how, now that she was a member of an elite trained group, she
had the world as her oyster.

Leavers and stayers: the first career decision
At Southampton Poor Law Infirmary 70% of entrants (317) to
training between 1902 and 1920 completed training; 185 then
immediately left the hospital with their various certificates.
Between 1895 and 1904 The London Hospital granted 796 certificates to trained nurses, of whom only 28% (224) stayed for any
length of time at the hospital after training.[16] Whether all
of these newly-certificated nurses left voluntarily or were
encouraged to leave is unclear but in reality this probably

amounted to the same thing. Nurses were positively encouraged
to leave their training hospital as early as possible -

> Human beings are like many plant forms; they require
> transplanting and in their early growth they thrive
> best in a not too thickly planted soil. It should
> take a few years to settle the question of her ulti-
> mate employ. Her destiny should not crystallize too
> soon. She should not allow herself to get planted
> too deep.[17]

Within the voluntary sector it was widely acknowledged
that most nurses would leave after qualifying; this practice
was also prevalent in the Poor Law hospitals after the turn
of the century;

> The question is often asked as to whether the nurses
> remain at the expiration of their training in the
> service of the Poor Law. And that a large number do
> seek other fields of labour appear to me to be a
> matter neither for astonishment nor regret. At the
> expiration of the 3 year training ... she is a free
> agent and should be encouraged in selecting the
> branch of nursing service most beneficial to herself.[18]

The hierarchical structure of hospital nursing was itself
responsible for many trained nurses seeking work outside of
the training hospital. The typical staff structure was that of
the Middlesex Hospital (1908), given in a guide to matrons -

> The distribution of the nursing staff must neces-
> sarily vary very much, according to the arrangement
> of wards, numbers of beds, class of cases, and off-
> duty time. Generally speaking, a proportion of one
> nurse to 3 patients, spread over the total number of
> beds, is a convenient one. This would work out at
> one-third of the total nursing staff on night-duty,
> and two thirds on day-duty, exclusive of Sisters.
>   There are usually 3 grades of nurses ... who
> may be roughly divided for a total of 100 into
>
> | | |
> |---|---|
> | 1st year probationers | 30 |
> | 2nd year probationers | 40 |
> | Staff Nurses | 30 |
> | | 100 |

These might be distributed in three's (one of each
grade) to wards of 20 beds, with an extra probationer to take 'time-off' and a staff nurse to each
ward on night duty and a probationer to help between
every two wards.[19]

In the Poor Law hospitals, with generally no out-patient departments to be staffed, the average proportion of nurses to patients in a well-staffed infirmary was 1 nurse to 8.5 patients.[20] Allowing that each ward was under the charge of a sister, the actual difference in staffing levels between the two sectors was manifest at the junior level, that is, among the probationer and staff nurses.

No matter how many trained nurses were produced annually, there were at the most only two or three qualified nurses required or employed per ward; most newly qualified nurses had no internal qualified post to go to and were obliged to leave or, in the case of the voluntary hospitals, to go onto the private staff of the hospital and await a suitable vacancy on a ward.

The isolation of the ward sister, as perhaps the only but always the most senior trained nurse on a ward, fulfilled the Nightingale - dictum of the centrality of this nursing grade. For Nightingale, the ward sister was "the true Mother of her ward" and the ward itself was her "home", and the patients her "family"; divided authority could only lead to a diminution of her role and status within the hospital infrastructure. Trained nurses had to leave, then, and those who were permitted to stay had to become sisters-in-training - staff nurses.[21]

A far more important, although largely unspoken, reason for the lack of high numbers of trained staff at the bedside was the potential cost which such a structure would mean to the hospital subscribers or local rate-payers. Table 4.1 outlines the relative salary costs of an actual nursing structure on an average ward compared with one of the many possible alternatives and Table 4.2 illustrates the costs of nursing to specific institutions. It is apparent that it was considerably cheaper to use probationers and that that was the case must say something about the nature of nursing skills actually needed, rather than occupationally argued for.[22]

Some trained nurses did stay in their training hospitals, however; during the earlier years of general hospital training, who stayed depended on the relationship between the individual nurse and her matron, particularly when the total number of nurses in training was small enough to allow personal and frequent contact between these grades. Such a network inevitably broke down as the number of probationers increased and as new nursing grades were inserted between the matron and the ward staff, such as the home sister, assistant matron and sister-tutor. Some method was needed whereby the matron could select individual nurses for praise, reward and promotion within the hospital. That method, a mimicry of the most easily available model - the medical school - involved giving prizes and medals, the most important of which were awarded at the end of training.[23]

Furnished with examination results and reports from ward sisters and other members of nursing's moral policeforce

Table 4.1: Cost per Ward of Nursing Salaries, Actual and Suggested Schemes (£'s per annum)

Grade	Actual				Suggested			
	1898		1927		1898		1927	
	Voluntary	Poor Law	Voluntary	Poor Law	Voluntary	Poor Law	Voluntary	Poor Law
Sister	30	28	75	75	30	28	70	75
Sister	–	–	–	–	30	28	70	75
Staff Nurse	24	22	55	60	24	22	55	60
Staff Nurse	–	–	–	–	24	22	55	60
Staff Nurse	–	–	–	–	24	22	55	60
Staff Nurse	–	–	–	–	24	22	55	60
3rd Year Prob.	19	18	30	40		(Supernumerary)		
2nd Year Prob.	13	14	25	35				
1st Year Prob.	11	8	20	30				
1st Year Prob.	–	–	–	–				
Totals	97	90	200	240	156	144	360	390

Source: H. C. Burdett, Burdett's Official Nursing Directory (Scientific Press, London, 1898).

Report by the Labour Party, The Labour Party and the Nursing Profession (Labour Party, London, 1927).

Table 4.2: Cost of Nurses during 1903 at Selected General Hospitals

Institution	Daily Ave. of Occupied Beds	Total Nursing Staff	% of 1st year Probationers on Staff	Average Cost of Maintenance per Head. £	Average Cost of Laundry per Head. £	Average Cost of Nurses of Nurses per Head. £
The London	676	395	37	21.5	6.5	52.25
Guys	499	261	(not known)	16	5.5 b	37
Barts	535	241	(not known)	16.5	4	47
St. Thomas's	442	165	27	23	5	56
St. George's	269	144	(not known)	17.5	5	52
Middlesex	312	138	41	21	5	45
St. Mary's	255	100	28	26	4	53
Kings College	184	81	(not known)	31	5	59
Univ. College	166	79	45	18.5 a	6	45
Charing Cross	137	61	24	(not known)	5	(not known)
Royal Free	145	50	24	20	6	51
Ave. London	329	156	32⅔	21	5.2	49.75
Birmingham	289	101	24	16.5	3	38
Sheffield	208	67	30	25	-2	47
Glasgow	441	151	26	26	-2	48
Ave. these 3	312⅔	106⅓	26⅔	22.5	3	44⅓

Source: Sir H.C. Burdett, Evidence, Select Committee on the Registration of Nurses (Parliamentary Papers, 1905). Appendix 6, p. 185 (abridged).

a. Average for 1902 given.
b. Hospital has its own private laundry.

- for example, the home sister - the matron or the Nursing
Committee was able to single out individuals as 'model' nurses
and award them medals and prizes. This elite could then be
selected to remain in the service of the hospital (on the
grounds that it was better to retain the best rather than the
average), or they could be offered further, specialised training or experience. Miss Wilson had the first choice offered to
her but turned it down -

> Bart's tried to persuade me to join their staff in
> any capacity I fancied - being a Gold Medalist, it
> was my duty to remain in the hospital and adorn
> the nursing staff, etc., etc. Not a bit of it! I
> was off to pastures new and, I hoped, to many ad-
> ventures.[24]

'Post-graduate' courses were taken within the training
hospital or in one which had close links with it: in this way
a particular specialism could be provided with a small but
continuous supply of 'superior' labour, and usually at a relatively low cost since many of these medalists and prize-win-
ners continued to receive only probationer rates of pay. An
additional bonus of this scheme was that the medalist was normally required to return to the general hospital for at least
the equivalent period that she had been away, thus ensuring a
ready supply of trained nurses for the training hospital to
draw upon. The system could never truly function absolutely as
Miss Wilson's case shows, since medalists were aware that they
were likely to get quick promotion by going elsewhere, but it
was the only way in which nursing was able to continue to
identify 'preferred' members of its own ranks.
  For those nurses who chose the institutional life, "whose
regularity and routine ... appealed to many characters", the
usual steps to promotion were from "probationer to Staff or
Charge Nurse, then in succession to Ward Sister, Night Superintendent, Home Sister and Matron's Assistant".[25]
  The staff nurse did "most of the actual nursing" by day
and night and took charge of the ward in the sister's absence.
Job descriptions for staff nurses did appear in the literature,
listing the many tasks performed by the grade of nurse: however, the ambiguous nature of the post, which could be held at
times by a senior probationer, at other times by trained and
certificated nurses suggests that few contemporaries saw in
the post anything other than a temporary, very temporary, step
on the path to becoming a sister.[26] Despite the high level of
patient-contact involved at this grade, the staff nurse was,
vide Nightingale, only a trained nurse en route to becoming a
training nurse, a ward sister.
  The articles and handbooks aimed at assisting the ward
sister in her duties are in marked contrast to the lack of
such advice for the staff nurse.[27] According to one such

source, "the post of Ward Sister is one of no small responsibility and influence, as many interests and duties must be considered, and an even balance maintained between them all."
[28] The ward sister was the key to the training of new nurses - through her "the trained matron influences nurses, probationers, ward maids and patients throughout the hospital" - and she had to balance the rival claims on her time, "her duty to her patients" and her duty as a teacher, to ensure the smooth functioning of the institution.[29] No wonder then her centrality, no wonder she is the figure most frequently recalled in nursing memoirs;[30] yet Hughes only _suggested_ experience as a ward sister to London-trained nurses before they sought a matronship - "an appointment, if only for a short time as a Sister of a ward is good experience" but not essential.[31]

Hughes' advice could only apply to a small select group even within this elite corps of trained general nurses; more realistic was her other suggestion, that a newly qualified nurse should "go in for extra certificates so soon as her engagement is over".[32] Such qualifications ranged from the fringe areas of fashionable medicine (swedish massage, gymnastics, hydrotherapy) to more popular mainstream experience, midwifery, massage, housekeeping and domestic management. For the nurse who had chosen the institutional life certificates such as these allowed her to compete for senior posts in the specialised areas of nursing as well as giving her opportunity to try for senior positions in general hospital nursing itself.

Further qualifications were another string to the bow of the certificated nurse opting for private work; when not attending a general case she could take a maternity one, perhaps at a higher salary. As long as the majority of women continued to give birth at home, the maternity- and midwife-nurse would find employment, but only the doubly-certificated nurse could ride out any period of under- or unemployment with comparative ease.

A certificate in midwifery was also a prerequisite for a number of non-nursing posts which attracted some hospital nurses as candidates, in particular the evolving occupation of health visiting. For those women "fond of foreign experiences" the C.M.B. certificate was an "absolute essential, for even though this certificate is not recognised in the Colonies to which the nurse is sent as being a guarantee of efficient training in midwifery, every nurse going abroad should be prepared to perform the duties of a midwife in an emergency."[33]

While there were training schemes in massage for nurses, there were none for areas of nursing newly developed, such as X-ray nursing, and few nurses thought about such areas of work as careers. More certificated nurses sought training and certification if possible in hospital management or housekeeping, since the possession of those skills could lead to senior nursing appointments, such as assistant matron, home sister

and matron's posts themselves.[34] Occasionally, housekeeping
training and certification could be obtained before nurse
training, which was a useful way of keeping hold of a recruit
who was debarred from beginning training on the grounds of
youth.[35]

The many certificates which the 'graduate' was able to
collect increased the range of expertise which the individual
nurse could offer, thus increasing her chances of obtaining
senior appointments in the hospital sectors. Since such further training normally took place immediately after qualifying as a general nurse, giving the general nurse no time to
practice or perfect the training she had received, those nurses who then sought and obtained senior posts in other institutions, despite being highly qualified 'on paper', had to
rely for their basic skills on experience as a general probationer. This was one of the reasons put forward by contemporaries for lengthening the training programme, but as we noted
at the beginning of this chapter, few felt that the trained
nurse ever lost anything once she had been properly trained.
This confidence in the universality of basic general training
helped the general nurse to overcome any personal reluctance
to enter specialised areas of nursing as well as overpowering
any misgivings which the specialised area personnel might have
harboured.[36]

Apart from the fact that most newly qualified nurses
were 'encouraged' to leave their training hospitals, the decisions made by graduates to follow particular career patterns depended as much on personal idiosyncrasies and attitudes as on the relative advantages and disadvantages which
particular branches of nursing may have offered. Mrs. Mc-
Lellan, for example, who trained towards the end of the First
World War, said that she had "wanted to join the army in
order to go abroad, but I was put off by having to wear the
uniform even to dances."[37]

Whatever the personal reasons given for a choice of career there were wide differences in conditions of service between institutional nursing, private nursing, nursing in the
Services and nursing posts abroad. The most insiduous was the
degree of personal freedom enjoyed by the woman: the most immediate and obvious distinction was the financial reward offered for the type of nursing performed. Tables 4.3 - 4.5
summarise the rates of pay in some of the major areas of nursing work in the period. The salary received varied not only
between Poor Law and voluntary hospitals, but between hospital
nursing and non-institutional areas of work. Most branches of
the work offered some form of board and lodging as well as the
basic salary or fee. In the hospitals the cost to the management - or benefit to the nurse - could equal if not exceed
the money wages paid. The total cost or value of board and
lodging, including maintenance, laundry and uniform, varied
between a high of £59 p.a. at King's College Hospital, London

Table 4.3: Annual Salaries paid to various grades of trained nurses 1870 - 1933, England and Wales, Voluntary Hospitals (in £'s)

Grade	1870 - 1899	1900 - 1909	1910 - 1919	1920 - 1933
General Hospitals				
Matron	- [a]	100 - 300	100 - 350	- [a]
Assistant Matron	- [a]	- [a]	60 - 70	- [a]
Superintendent of Nurses	- [a]	- [a]	120 - 150	- [a]
Night Superintendent	- [a]	- [a]	- [a]	- [a]
Home Sister	- [a]	- [a]	- [a]	- [a]
Ward Sister	26 - 35	30 - 50	78 - 120	65 - 130
Staff Nurse	20 - 30	20 - 30	64 - 80	28 - 90
Hospital Private Nurse	25 - 40	- [a]	80 - 95	55 - 80

Sources: Sir H. C. Burdett, Burdett's Official Directory of Nurses (Scientific Press, London, 1898), pp. 36-90.
L. Maule, 'Training Schools and Other Nursing Institutions' in (various authors), Science and Art of Nursing (Cassells, London, 1908), pp. 46-93.
H. Todd, 'Nursing in Poor Law Institutions in England and Wales' in (various authors), Science and Art of Nursing (Cassells, London, 1908), pp. 128-48.
Women's Employment, 7 January 1910.
Sir H. C. Burdett, How to Succeed as a Trained Nurse (Scientific Press, London, 1913), pp. 10-23.
W. Whittall, Pensions for Hospital Officers and Staffs (Layton, London, 1919), p. 208.
Sir H. C. Burdett, How To Become a Nurse (Faber and Faber, London, 1933).
A. Chapman, Studies in the National Income and Expenditure of the United Kingdom: Volume 5: Wages and Salaries in the United Kingdom 1920 - 1933 (C.U.P., Cambridge, 1953), p. 202.
G. M. Ayers, England's First State Hospitals 1867 - 1930 (Wellcome, London, 1971), p. 333.
F. F. Waddy, A History of Northampton General Hospital 1743 - 1948 (Guildhall, London, 1974), p. 148.
R. White, Social Change and the Development of the Nursing Profession (Kimpton, London, 1978), p. 170

a. Not available or no comparable grade.

126

Table 4.4: Annual Salaries paid to various grades of trained nurses 1870 - 1933, England and Wales, Poor Law Hospitals (in £'s)

Grade	1870 - 1899	1900 - 1909	1910 - 1919	1920 - 1933
General Hospitals				
Matron	- [a]	100 - 150	45 - 150	150 - 500
Assistant Matron	- [a]	40 - 60	40 - 60	100 - 230
Superintendent of Nurses	- [a]	- [a]	- [a]	- [a]
Night Superintendent	35	35 - 45	40 - 60	110 - 135
Home Sister	- [a]	30 - 40	40 - 60	100 - 160
Ward Sister	30	26 - 35	28 - 40	85 - 125
Staff Nurse	15 - 30	22	30 - 35	60 - 80
Hospital Private Nurse	- [a]	- [a]	- [a]	- [a]

Sources: As Table 4.3
a. As Table 4.3

Table 4.5: Annual salaries paid to various grades of trained nurses 1870 - 1933, England and Wales, Fever and Mental Hospitals (in £'s)

	1870 - 1899	1900 - 1909	1910 - 1919	1920 - 1933
Fever Hospitals				
Matron	75 - 120	100 - 150	- [a]	160 - 340
Ward Sister	27	36 - 40	- [a]	80 - 95
Staff Nurse	- [a]	30 - 34	- [a]	60 - 70
Mental Hospitals				
Matron	150 - 200	100 - 150	- [a]	240 - 340
Ward Sister	30 - 40	33 - 43	40 - 100 [b]	96 - 128
Staff Nurse	- [a]	25 - 31	40 - 100 [b]	94 - 114

Sources: As Table 4.3
a. As Table 4.3
b. Between 1910 - 1919 the following rates of salary were earnt by the respective non-hospital nurses: Self-employed Private Nurse £36 - £60; Nursing Institute Private Nurse £26 - £30; Co-operative Private Nurse £80 - £100; Private Mental Nurse £80 - £90; Village Nurse £50 - £70; Midwifery and Monthly Nurse £25 - £100. Sources: As Table 4.3.

and a low of £37 p.a. at Guy's Hospital, London, with a mean average for London of £49.75 (1903).[38]

Certificated nurses working outside of hospitals received board and lodging from their employer, private or agency. A minority did not get such allowances and may have preferred to be 'non-resident'. The willingness of some nurses to provide private care on a daily or visiting basis was a new development in this period in response to and in an attempt to compete with the private staff of the voluntary hospitals.

The opportunities open to certificated nurses and the conditions under which she worked were many and varied, from the statutory terms of engagement in the Poor Law hospitals, through the rules and statutes of the individual voluntary hospital to the vagaries of the self-employed market. While we cannot be precise about the phenomena now called "labour turnover" for the period 1881 - 1914, we can provide a series of descriptions of typical career patterns, which will complement the discussion of pre-nursing experiences and allow some generalisations to be made about the role nursing may have played in geographical, occupational and social mobility.

A series of typical nursing careers

A recent discussion (1979) of the employment of nurses within the National Health Service has suggested that trained nurses are "an essentially short-service group who are highly mobile in the early years after qualification", but whose movement is normally within the National Health Service.[39] Trained nurses moving between hospitals do so, according to that research, not out of dislike of their old employers, but out of a "commitment to Nursing", since the moves were made because of "the 'pull' of another institution, or the promotion it is perhaps offering, rather than the 'push' of dissatisfying circumstances in their present hospital".Nursing labour turnover is a "social process" in which a certain amount of mobility is regarded as "normal and beneficial", both for nurses and for the employer, the National Health Service.[40]

As we have noted, few newly-qualified nurses stayed in their training hospitals and while there were some economic advantages attached to particular forms of nursing work, these were not the most significant factor in causing that mobility. The pull of promotion, whether achieved or not, served as a stronger force in drawing nurses into post-basic training or into other hospitals, even if they were smaller than the nurse was used to. Even where this pull was transformed, as in private nursing, into the degree of freedom of action in professional and personal life, it was this and not the material rewards which drew the nurses out of the hospitals.

The major push factor in contemporary turnover was undoubtedly the burden of costs which a high ratio of trained nurses entailed, at a time when it appeared that there was a growing demand for probationer posts. Whether that mobility was beneficial to nursing and medical care in toto is questionable; it is more certain that it benefitted many individual nurses, and enhanced the role of general hospital nursing in the hierarchy of the occupation. We can examine that process by looking at a series of typical careers for general hospital trained nurses; these may be divided into (a) those who stayed in the training institution; (b) those who remained within their original training sector - Poor Law or voluntary - even if they took additional training; (c) those who joined the ranks of private nursing, and (d) those who moved between Poor Law and voluntary hospitals but who stayed in the general sector.

The first pattern, as we have noted, was probably the least common and depended on examination success and the medal system then in vogue. Retention by the training hospital inevitably meant promotion, sometimes immediately on qualifying - Emma Bayliss spent 1882 - 1883 as a probationer at the Nightingale School and was promoted sister on completion of her probationary year. This happened in other voluntary hospitals, and not just in the London ones; for example -

Grace	Lady probationer	)		1882-83
Benson	Sister (Accident Ward)	)	Guy's	1883-84
	Sister (Stephen Ward)	)	Hospital	1884-85
	Night Sister	)		1885-89
Adelaide	Probationer	)	Royal	1886-87
Chalker	Staff Nurse	)	Infirmary	1887-89
	Sister	)	Halifax	1889-98
Lucy	Probationer	)	Birmingham	1893-96
Duval	Sister	)	Gen. Hosp.	1896-98

Such promotion was also found in the Poor Law sector, although for less nurses because of fewer hospitals actually training nurses; for example

Kate	Probationer	)	Brownlow	1880-81
Kearney	Staff Nurse	)	Hill	1881-83
	Matron	)	Infirmary	1883-85
Lydia	Probationer	)		1879-80
Twanley	Staff Nurse	)	Crumpsall	1880-82
	Sister	)	Infirmary	1882-85
				41

Some of these 'non-movers' spent their entire working lives in the one institution, as Mr. Todd confirmed to the Select Committee on Metropolitan Hospitals (1890) - "head nurses stop a long time. We have one head nurse who has been in the service of the hospital now for about 20 years; another head nurse who has been in the hospital about 18 years."[42]

The second pattern shows the nurse remaining in her original training sector, Poor Law or voluntary. Official explanations spoke of the social problems which faced the voluntary-hospital trained nurse descending to the level of the Poor Law service, in particular the waste of her talents, while the trained nurse moving the other way was faced, it was argued, with a lack of acute nursing experience needed in the voluntary hospitals. The strict spheres of responsibility in the Poor Law service, between nurses and the Masters and Matrons, nurses and the Boards of Guardians, and nurses and the Medical Superintendents, were seen by contemporaries to be potential sources of conflict of power and authority for the new voluntary-hospital trained nurse, as were the assumed differences in social status between voluntary-hospital nurses and Poor Law patients and, indeed, Poor Law doctors.[43]

As we have noted, the social origins of recruits to each sector were not so distinct as contemporary accounts suggest, which assumes that it was training in a voluntary hospital, and not origin, which conferred nursing status. When the Metropolitan Asylums Board attempted to find out why few trained nurses were being attracted to the Poor Law infirmaries, they discovered that it was not the salary differences which were to blame: the main reason given by the nurses themselves was that the official title in the Poor Law service for the nurse in charge of a ward was "charge nurse" and that this title "mitigated against their getting sister's posts afterwards by not being able to quote the fact of 'sister-ships' against applicants from voluntary hospitals".[44]

There was a more important reason for the non-movement of nurses between the two sectors than that of title, albeit the significance of such matters to nurses; while nurses were working they were being paid and kept by the hospital, when they ceased to work, due to age or sickness, they stopped being supported by the institution.

Nurses in the Poor Law hospitals had had no pension rights until they were included in the Poor Law Superannuation Act (Revised) 1897, and long-serving nurses often found themselves ill-equipped to face retirement or protracted sickness. After the Act, those nurses who did not opt out of the contributory scheme could receive a reasonable sum per annum when retired, provided they had been employed in the service for the required number of years. A charge nurse (ward sister) retiring aged 65 years, with more than ten years service at that grade received a pension of about £65 p.a. by 1910, when her salary and emoluments may have been valued at approximately £100 p.a.[45]

Voluntary hospital nurses looked on this pension scheme with some envy, seeing in it "an immense boon to nurses" everywhere.[46] The voluntary hospital nurse had three options as far as retirement was concerned; ignore the problem and/or perhaps save piecemeal for themselves; rely on the goodwill and charity of an employer or hospital Committee; or contribute to a private pension scheme, such as The Royal National Pension Fund for Nurses, set up in 1887 through the efforts of Sir Henry Burdett.[47]

Individual voluntary hospitals rewarded long service with a pension or gratuity, although they were under no obligation to do so. Some hospitals had elaborate schemes, such as that at Bart's where in 1908 the pension amounted to two-thirds of the annual salary and emoluments for nurses with a minimum of 36 years service, although a smaller pension could be granted from the age of 55 years.[48] Before the turn of the century, nurses at the Royal Infirmary, Manchester, appear to have had to petition for a pension, which varied according to length of service - "Sister Catherine Gaynor applied for a pension on completion of 25 years service, and being over 50 years of age and unfit to work, she was granted a pension of £25 p.a."[49]

By 1916 most voluntary hospitals provided a pension for retiring nurses, most but not all affiliated to the R.N.P.F.N: a contemporary report on nurses' pensions noted, however, that many nurses postponed their retirement beyond the minimum allowed "until actual ill-health renders further service impossible".[50] This was not out of altruism, but was evidence of the "hardship resulting from the inadequate provision of pensions"[51] and an earlier commentator had pointed out that many nurses failed to receive pensions, or only small ones, because of broken service.[52] One major advantage which the R.N.P.F.N. scheme set out to provide from its inception was the carrying over of pension contributions, thus allowing the "migration of nurses" between hospitals, between sectors and even between institutional and non-institutional work.[53] Few nurses, however, seem to have taken real advantage of this remarkable improvement in their conditions of service, despite the initial success of the R.N.P.F.N; indeed, most nurses would have agreed with Mrs. O'Keefe when she said "I never made plans for a pension. No, I was one of those 'live-todays'".[54]

Among those nurses who stayed in their training sector were those who had several posts early in their careers; some of these were no doubt obtaining nursing experiences missing from their original training which were considered necessary for 'all-round' competence, either by taking another training or spending a few weeks or months in a specialised hospital.

The most numerically significant area of nursing in the period up to the First World War was private nursing. Burdett estimated that there were just over 11,000 female nurses working in hospitals in 1903, out of a total nursing population of approximately 55,000: in other words, and allowing for other areas of nursing work, nearly 70% of all "bona fide" nurses up to 1914 were working in the private sector.[55]

Contemporaries were well aware of the high proportion of private nurses: reformers like the Fenwicks made it clear that the prime motive for State Registration was to ensure the provision of trained nurses for private cases.[56] However, the take-over of private nursing by the hospital-trained nurse was not completely welcome; Miss Todd thought that "the more or less mechanical training in hospital was responsible for the rigidity of the average nurse. In hospital, nurses were necessarily trained for institution work, on somewhat mechanical lines: patients were expected to do, and usually did, exactly as they were told; this did not tend to develop the tactful initiative so necessary in dealing with patients who did not expect to obey in detail."[57]

The self-styled "first historian of Nursing in Great Britain", Sarah Tooley, described private nursing as the most lucrative branch of the profession and pointed out that hospital matrons were complaining by the turn of the century that they were "constantly losing good nurses who are attracted by the freer life and better chances for making money which private nursing offers."[58] It was a career for those who looked for "new places" and new faces, but one which offered complete success only to "the best type of nurse", echoing the Fenwickian anxieties about unqualified women practising as nurses.

Private nurses had three avenues of employment; through their own efforts; by working for an agency or institution supplying private nurses, or by joining a co-operative. The independent private nurse had at least two advantages over other private nurses - she could set her own fees, leaving it up to the 'market' to determine whether she was employed or not; she could set herself up as a private nurse irrespective of hospital training or experiences. The first advantage, perhaps because it was more apparent than real, was hardly mentioned in the common attacks on the independent operator by the pro-Registrationists, the second was a continual source of annoyance to the trained nurse.

Many private nurses working on their own account relied on word-of-mouth recommendation by doctors or ex-patients, or set themselves up in an area where they then hoped to become known. This 'localisation' had been a source of annoyance to some voluntary hospitals even before they set up their own private nursing departments. Nurses leaving the employ of such hospitals were required to sign an undertaking not to practise within a given area, usually 3 miles from the hospital, but as often within an even wider area. These restrictions became less necessary and less applied as the voluntary hospitals entered the private practice field and thus increased their domination of the private patient market.[59]

Other private nurses advertised their availability in the general press, popular magazines such as The Lady or in the nursing journals themselves.[60] Just as the governess had discovered,[61] the potential employers of private nurses were increasingly reluctant to engage a resident nurse, either on grounds of lack of accommodation, a growing discomfort felt by the middle-class around servants in general, or by the costs which were involved in such service.[62] The average independent private nurses could expect to earn 2 guineas per week plus board and lodging for a general case and 3 guineas for a maternity case (1898), and from the end of the century some began to offer a visiting daily service to patients. This meant that such women could now perhaps marry and still practise, and after the 1890's the practice forced the private nursing agencies to take up daily care in order to compete with the undercutting independent operator.

For those private nurses lacking initiative or local knowledge, or unprepared to accept periods of unemployment and hence no income, the agencies and co-operatives offered more security. The first nursing agencies had been closely tied to religious groups;[63] however, the Mildmay Institution was a temperance society and one of the first non-sectarian private associations providing trained private nurses to the public (1868). It and the many which followed its example undertook to train women in general hospitals providing they agreed to continue in the service of the institution for at least three years.[64] Co-operatives extended the management of the agencies to the nurses themselves through elections to the management committee, the first appearing in 1891, although many were far from being true co-operative ventures in reality.

A period spent as a private nurse did not debar the certificated nurse from returning to hospital work, confirming contemporary statements about the "longevity" of the original probationer training. Mary Holland spent 4 years as a private nurse before returning to become a ward sister at the West Herts. Infirmary, Hemel Hempstead (1896); Julia Moule returned to hospital work in 1892 after three years as a private and district nurse in London; Clare Rogers became a head nurse at Cuckfield Union Infirmary in 1895 having trained in a voluntary hospital and a Poor Law fever hospital, and after 4 years as an independent private nurse.[65]

A final career pattern may be identified from contemporary sources - the movement between voluntary and Poor Law hospitals, (see above, however). Writing in 1913 Burdett advised the newly qualified voluntary-hospital nurse to "pass into the Poor Law Service, and take up sisterships or administrative posts", although he also warned his readers that since the training in the Poor Law hospitals had so improved, the ease with which they could make that move was becoming restricted.[66]

In the early years of the Poor Law nursing service, which owed its impetus to the Order of 1887,[67] it was unremarkable that voluntary-hospital trained nurses should find senior posts in the Poor Law hospitals; there were simply not enough Poor Law trained nurses available. By the outbreak of War it was not only providing for its own needs but actually adding to the 'surplus' of trained nurses in the country.[68] Despite

this development, voluntary-hospital trained nurses continued
to be appointed to many of the vacancies at senior level in
the Poor Law sector.

Of the 70 or so voluntary-hospital trained nurses registered with Burdett in 1898 and then working in the Poor Law
sector, almost half were in assistant matron or matron posts,
and only ten in junior or staff nurse posts. Miss E. Price was
trained for one year at Guy's Hospital, 1889-90; she then
spent six years as a ward sister at Guy's before being appointed Matron of Mill Road Infirmary, Liverpool a Poor Law hospital of 850 beds. The first superintendent matron and head
nurse of the Leeds Union Infirmary (1899) was Miss Joanna
Hopper, a graduate of The London Hospital, 1888-91, who had
had two years experience as a ward sister at The Taunton and
Somerset Hospital and nine months experience as a matron of a
cottage hospital.[69]

Occasionally senior appointments in a Poor Law hospital
were held by successive graduates of one or other voluntary
hospital, the case at Leeds Infirmary between 1894 and c1910.
At other times the matron and assistant matron posts were held
by nurses trained in the same hospital and, indeed, it was not
thought unusual in the closing years of the nineteenth-century
for trained nurses to follow specific matrons into new hospitals. Whether this was due to personal ties of friendship,
patronage or a need to bask in 'reflected glory' is unclear;
it does, however, show how readily voluntary-hospital trained
nurses moved into the Poor Law sector.

It would not be going too far beyond the data to suggest
that much of this mobility from voluntary to Poor Law hospitals was due to the ease with which promotion and higher salaries could be obtained by such nurses. With the exception of
the 'exceptions' i.e. those medalists etc. who stayed on in
their training schools, voluntary nurses were promoted more
quickly into the Poor Law sector than other nurses, as Burdett
had tacitly acknowledged in his advice to trained nurses cited
earlier.

There remains one other career pattern which needs to be
discussed before we can leave the subject of career choices
in nursing: that pattern takes account of those certificated
nurses who left the occupation after qualifying, often without
ever working as a trained nurse at all.

By its very nature as a 'non-career', it is almost impossible to discover personal motives for leaving nursing, nor is
it possible to know with any precision just how many nurses
left at that stage. Nursing records tend to limit themselves
to those who trained and to those who remained, and only
rarely comment on why certificated (as opposed to in-training)
nurses left altogether. There can be none of the exactitude of
Mercer's recent study into nursing labour turnover, which included in its findings that nursing work shares equally the
"source of personal growth and social relationships" with

family life.[70] For the hospital nurse at the beginning of the twentieth-century such equality was impossible because of a marriage bar; those who wanted "the combination of raising/ looking after a family and working" were forced out of the hospitals and into the private sector.[71] Despite the popularity of this sector, however, the numbers of private nurses listed in Burdett's register (1898) and who were married was less than 100 out of a total of 4,000 trained nurses. Only 2% of trained nurses who might wish to combine work and family life seem to have done so, and some of these must have been widows who needed to work; either the combination was unworkable or, more likely, those who wished to marry gave up nursing entirely.

Some nurses made the step from nursing to nursing-and-marriage via private work; a few via lectureships in Hygiene, Nursing (i.e. home nursing), massage and so on, and a very small number via the ownership of nursing agencies, health visiting or posts as lady sanitary inspectors. For many more, however, there was no such step, either because a marriage bar existed in many occupations open to them or because work and marriage was not ideologically acceptable to women and men in the social class in which nurses found themselves.

The origins of the marriage bar in nursing lie in the Appendix to the Notes on Nursing (3rd edition, 1863) written by Florence Nightingale, and as such bear testimony to the strength and pervasiveness of her influence on nursing in the ensuing 50 years. In her review of contemporary systems of nursing, Nightingale formulated the principle that nurses should be single women because "married women (are) no longer attached to (their) work but to (their) husbands". No woman could serve two hearths; she must either be the good-woman-nurse or the good-woman-wife.[72] The principle was eagerly taken up by other reformers, including Dr. Swete the propagandist of the cottage hospital system:[73] however, such statements about the value of married women as nurses were mere rhetoric, as Nightingale herself acknowledged: if she was called upon to prove her case, she could only do so by quoting "instances of such gross physical or moral neglect (though generally unintentional) that it would be useless to enter on such a crusade."[74]

The marriage bar, based on polemic, owed much to the demographic changes in the mid- and late-Victorian periods, notably the changing sex ratio and the chances of marriage for women. Similar arguments based on the 'surplus women problem' were found in the movements towards a marriage bar in teaching and even in domestic service.[75] The consequences of the operation of a bar for nursing were the even closer association of nursing with womanhood, the substitution or the interchangeability of tasks, duties, obligations and commitments between the two spheres and, (as in teaching) a proportionate loss of trained and certificated women from the occupation at the

earliest opportunity.[76] But as Miss Stansfield reassured the
Select Committee investigating the operation of the Poor Laws
(1909), as long as the supply of probationers never ran dry,
even if they stayed only a short time, any change in nursing
was only likely to be towards the standardisation and evening-
up between Poor Law and voluntary sectors, and not to any fundamental questioning of underlying assumptions or practices.
She might have added, though she did not, that as long as
single women needed 'respectable' work married women would be
forcibly kept out of general hospital nursing.[77]

Conclusion
For the woman who had been through a course of nurse training,
be it one year as a lady pupil at a prestigious London voluntary hospital or three years at a 'recognised' Poor Law infirmary, a certificate as a trained general nurse offered many
opportunities by which she might earn a living and perhaps,
given her reduced chances of marriage, support herself in retirement and old age. The structure of contemporary nursing,
which ranged from the one-to-one, employer/employee relationship of private nursing, through the control of small cottage
hospitals and sanatoria to the senior positions in large Poor
Law and voluntary general hospitals, allowed the certificated
nurse an ever-increasing occupational career choice.
    The basis upon which such choices were made not only re-
flected personal motive, ambition and character of the woman
making them but also the very structure of the world of nursing. There was prestige in being a ward sister in a hospital
with its own medical school and in being known as "Sister
Victor" or "Sister Opthalmic".[78] There was an additional filip
to be called 'matron' even if the post was one in charge of a
six-bedded cottage hospital or a hostel for homeless girls.
Amy Terton summed up her ambitions in her autobiography -

> So I used to think longingly of a cottage hospital as
> a place where there would be no probationers to train
> - a prospect that seemed bliss indeed. Gradually,
> when things went wrong, I got into a way of thinking,
> such a thing will not happen when I get my cottage
> hospital, till to be the Matron of one became the
> height of my ambition, and after a time the climax
> came.[79]

    For some nurses, close contact between the professional
and her clientele, as in private or district work, could satisfy the need of many contemporary nurses for social recognition and status.[80] This need could also be manifested as a
missionary zeal and translated into action by moving from voluntary to Poor Law sector. Such women were seen to be fulfilling Nightingale's wish that the trained nurse should train
others, take the new nursing order to those institutions lack-

136

ing progressive attitudes to nursing care and nursing roles.
The early 'nightingales' had done just that, although the
practice of sending St. Thomas-trained nurses out to hospitals in need of reform and trained nurses came to an end when
that illustrious hospital caught up with the twentieth-century
and put its trained nurses onto its own private staff co-operative and thus charged for their services (1908).[81]

The ideal of the new nurse as missionary remained in the
literature which urged voluntary hospital nurses to move into
the Poor Law sector. While it might have been an attempt to
influence the 'progress' of the Poor Law service, it was also
a useful means of shedding surplus and costly trained nurses.
The compensation offered for being a pioneer nurse and having
to face perhaps the scorn of friends at the decision was "the
mere fact of 'something attempted, something done', seeing
gradually a higher tone creeping over the whole place."[82]

The voluntary hospital nurse could influence the tone of
the Poor Law ward and hospital and even instil some manners
and respect for nursing and nurses into the Poor Law patients;
[83] she could more importantly transform the system of nursing
and the standard of care given in such hospitals. The pioneer
could take satisfaction "in seeing the nurses take a keen interest in their work, both theoretical and practical" after
she had taken charge. The new nurse could also reduce "the
heart-rending death-rate" found in these hospitals by her new
and skilled regime of nursing.[84] One such missionary ended her
account of the Poor Law service and the need for more voluntary hospital trained nurses to go into the work by saying

> One cannot have too high-class a nurse for infirmary
> nursing. There is so much a nurse with ideals can do,
> if she is broad-minded and sympathetic ... Oh, there
> is much in workhouse infirmary nursing that counts,
> and I hope girls and women of the right sort will
> not be deterred from entering. There is still a future
> before it, especially when the infirmaries are opened
> up to medical students, as I hope some day they will [85]
> be.

Miss Landale had argued for much the same in an article
written ten years earlier (1894); the pioneer should never
despair, she wrote, even "if the way is long, the ground rough
and perplexing" - that was after all why she was there in the
Poor Law - behind her in support was "the great army of Nurses,
who in the future will tend the sick poor in the workhouse infirmaries".[86]

There was resistance to the transfer of values from voluntary to Poor Law sectors, although much of the evidence for
it comes from the reformers and pioneers themselves as they
warned others of the pitfalls of infirmary nursing.[87] Antago-
nism to the new regime came not only from the existing Poor

Law nurses who tended to be lumped together as 'untrained assistant nurses' in such reports, but also from the Boards of Guardians, Poor Law medical officers and from some Poor Law patients themselves.

Overcoming this backward behaviour was what made the nurse a pioneer; her presence created the problem which only her presence could cure, so she was cautioned to walk on eggs and treat the Poor Law people, doctors, administrators and patients, as she would have her own hospital consultants and acquaintances.[88] As far as the Poor Law nurses were concerned, she was advised to continually watch them, never trusting them to do anything she had ordered, never expecting them to perform even routine tasks with any degree of skill let alone feeling of service to others;[89] the pioneer had to overcome the social habits of such women as were employed by the Poor Law authorities; as Landale recalled

> I cannot hope to make anyone realise how much I suffered at times during that period. The rudeness at first, of some of the nurses, their manners at table, their sneers at what they called 'the lady nurse'. One could not trust them to do their work conscienciously - temperatures habitually charted wrongly and nursing matters slurred over ... Still, some of the nurses were quite nice girls and willing and eager to learn their work properly.[90]

Such patience, perseverance and stoicism was supposed to be as effective in dealings with the Poor Law patients. Although the social distinction between voluntary and Poor Law patient was felt to be diminishing, the conditions from which the Poor Law patient was said to be suffering were still described as "chronic and tedious (sic)".[91] The voluntary hospital nurse who devoted herself to caring for such unfortunates could only extend the range of her own skills by nursing "such severe medical and heavy chronic cases",[92] skills she could then 'sell in the private nursing sector; such a nurse could also teach the poor sick to help themselves not only to better health, but through example and moral rectitude to break out of the cycle of pauperism and its attendant physical disease.[93]

The role of the voluntary nurse, and by extension the general nurse, as proselyte was well developed in the literature and she became portrayed as the bringer of a new order of nursing and a pioneer for civilisation itself:

> Attendance upon the sick, when pursued in the right spirit, is not only one of the noblest callings for man (i.e. doctor) or woman, but is, in its educational effects upon the individual, one of the most purifying and ennobling moral disciplines to which a human being can be subjected.

The true nurse, knowing her work and loving
it, has an individual force and attraction for
everybody which directly inspires confidence and
indirectly carries with it a moral influence for
good upon all whom her life may touch. This influence in the course of her nursing career, though
unknown to herself, sheds blessings which frequently
endure throughout the lifetime of the majority of
those who come within the spheres of her influence.[94]

A clearer expose of contemporary social imperialism and
social darwinist thought applied to the role of the nursing
profession may not be found;[95] the nurse was an agent of
social as much as physical reform. While the number of women
who chose to become pioneers for civilisation may have been
small, the consequences for the occupation were out of all proportion to their size. Even those nurses from 'lowly origins',
provided they obtained a certificate in general nursing, pre-
ferably though not necessarily from a prestigious voluntary
hospital, would advance in the occupation and have the opportunity to become pioneers.

Not all contemporary nurses took advantage of this opportunity, because it was less real than it appeared, but for
those who did, even partially, Goodrich's point about the uniform wiping out social distinctions is well vindicated by an
analysis of the post-certification career choices made by hospital-trained nurses. Within the occupation the general nurse
reigned supreme; what others outside of nursing, their potential clientele and their competitors, thought about their
claims to supremacy forms part of the next chapter.

NOTES

1. Goodrich, Significance of Nursing, p. 45.
2. Evidence of Lady Munro-Ferguson, Select Committee on
Registration of Nurses, 1905, vii, p. 132. See also, Nightingale, 'Training of Nurses', p. 236; Evidence of Miss Stewart,
Select Committee on Registration of Nurses, 1904, vi, p. 19;
G. Mercer, The Employment of Nurses: Nursing Labour Turnover in
the National Health Service (Croom Helm, London, 1979), p. 150.
3. Evidence of Dr. Moore, Select Committee on Registration of Nurses, 1904, vi, p. 49; Holland, Registration of
Nurses, 1904, p. 70.
4. Evidence of Sir J. Crichton-Browne, Select Committee
on Registration of Nurses, 1905, vii, p. 50.
5. Abel-Smith, Nursing Profession, p. 250. See also, Carpenter, 'Managerialism and Professionalism', p. 169; Carter,
New Deal, p. 71; Vivian, Lectures, p. 10.
6. For an introduction to the literature on nursing and
professionalisation see, Davies, 'Professionalizing Strategies',
pp. 1-10. See also, Reader, Professional Men; G. Millerson,

The Qualifying Associations: A Study in Professionalization
(Routledge and Kegan Paul, London, 1964); Holcombe, Victorian
Ladies at Work; P. V.Meyer, 'Professionalism and Social
Change in Rural Teachers in Nineteenth-Century France', Journal of Social History, June 1976, p. 545.
    7. Reader, Professional Men, p. 181; A. Etzioni, (edi-
tor), Semi-Professions and Their Organisation (Free Press, New
York, 1969).
    8. For an overview see, Abel-Smith, Nursing Profession,
Chapters V - VII; R. White, 'Some Political Influences surrounding the Nurses Registration Act 1919 in the United Kingdom', Journal of Advanced Nursing, 1, 1976, pp. 209-17. A
general discussion of the role of the State in women's 'white-
blouse' work is given by A. Grant, Socialism and the Middle
Classes (Laurence and Wishart, London, 1958).
    9. Abel-Smith, Nursing Profession, pp. 68-9.
    10. Ibid., pp. 68-9; Barritt, 'Nightingale's Values', pp.
26-30.
    11. Abel-Smith, Nursing Profession, pp. 68-9.
    12. Holland, Registration of Nurses, 1904, p. 32; Bur-
dett, Registration of Nurses, 1905, p. 109. See also, Evidence
of Miss Shannon, Select Committee on Registration of Nurses,
1905, vii, p. 124.
    13. Mrs. Kenwell, 'Oral evidence'; Mrs. McLellan, 'Oral
evidence'; Mrs. O'Keefe, 'Oral evidence'.
    14. Peterson, Medical Profession in London, Chapter IV.
    15. Holland, Registration of Nurses, 1904, p. 32; Bur-
dett, Registration of Nurses, 1905, p. 106; L.Seymer, Florence
Nightingale's Nurses: The Nightingale Training School 1860 -
1960, (Pitman, London, 1960), p. 109.
    16. Hospital Records; Evidence of Miss Luckes, Select
Committee on Registration of Nurses, 1905, vii. p. 172.
    17. R. O. Beard, 'The Social Development of the Nurse',
American Journal of Nursing, July 1912, p. 788.
    18. Stansfield, Poor Laws, 1909, p. 502. See also, Sey-
mer, Nightingale's Nurses, pp. 114-6.
    19. Vernet, 'Hospital Management', p. 117.
    20. Ibid., p. 129.
    21. Nightingale, 'Training of Nurses' p. 235; Seymer,
Nightingale's Nurses, p. 94.
    22. Smith, People's Health, pp. 280-84; Peterson, Medical
Profession in London, p. 138, p. 228; Woodward, To Do The Sick
No Harm, pp. 17-22; Carter, New Deal, p. 48, p. 57, p. 66, pp.
240-41; 'The Salaries of Nurses', British Journal of Nursing,
15 January 1921, p. 1. The cheapness of probationer labour is
discussed in Abel-Smith, Nursing Profession, pp. 228 et seq.,
and of student labour in general in Hogg, 'Employment', pp.
265-9.
    23. 'The Department of Modern Nursing', The Hospital, 11
August 1914, p. 418; Peterson, Medical Profession in London,
Chapter II; Brockbank, M.R.I., p. 62.

24. Wilson, Gone with the Raj, p. 15. See also, Hughes, 'Vocation', p. 100; 'The Hospital World: Some Bristol Hospitals', British Journal of Nursing, 8 June 1912, pp. 455-6.

25. Hughes, 'Vocation', pp. 98-9.

26. Ibid., p. 99; 'The Department of Modern Nursing', The Hospital, 30 May 1914, p. 247; 'The Department of Modern Nursing', The Hospital, 13 March 1913, p. 542. See also, Carter, New Deal, pp. 60-5; Laurence, Nurse's Life, Chapters XII - XVI.

27. For example, E. Luckes, Hospital Sisters and Their Duties (Churchill, London, 1886); Meadows, 'Ward Sister's Day'. The four volume Science and Art of Nursing (Cassells, London, 1908), was specifically for the trained ward sister.

28. Hughes, 'Vocation', p. 99.

29. Nightingale, 'Training of Nurses', p. 236; Seymer, Nightingale's Nurses, p. 89; Terton, Lights and Shadows, p. 70; Carpenter, 'Managerialism and Professionalism', pp. 178-89.

30. On occasion vying for popularity with 'great' doctors: see, for example, Brook, Nursing, pp. 7-8.

31. Hughes, 'Vocation', p. 100.

32. Ibid., p. 100.

33. Vivian, Lectures, pp. 93-4.

34. 'The Department of Modern Nursing', The Hospital, 8 August 1914, p. 531; Hughes, 'Vocation', p. 100.

35. Mrs. McLellan, 'Oral evidence'.

36. 'Reaction against progress', Nursing Mirror, 13 February 1909, p. 299.

37. Mrs. McLellan, 'Oral evidence'.

38. Burdett, Registration of Nurses, 1905, p. 185; see also, Abel-Smith, Nursing Profession, p. 280.

39. Mercer, Labour Turnover, p. 89.

40. Ibid., p. 9, p. 113. See also, Beard, 'Development', p. 788.

41. Burdett, Directory, 1898.

42. Evidence of Mr. Todd, Select Committee on the Metropolitan Hospitals, 1890/1, xiii, p. 102. See also, Brockbank, M. R. I., p. 61, p. 69.

43. Stansfield, Poor Laws, 1909, pp. 614-5; Burdett, Succeed, pp. 10-11; Landale, 'Workhouse Infirmary', pp. 6-8; C. Wood, 'The Present Position of Poor Law Nursing', Nursing Times, 10 June 1905, p. 91; 'Poor Law Nursing: The Nursing and Midwifery Conference', British Journal of Nursing, 3 May 1913, pp. 356-7; C. B. Wilkie, 'The Best Means of Providing and Training Nurses for the Indoor Poor', Nursing Record and Hospital World, 4 March 1899, p. 171; White, Social Change, pp. 78-93; Abel-Smith, Nursing Profession, pp. 45-9.

44. 'Shortage of Nurses', Nursing Times, 3 November 1907, p. 1035; 'The Shortage of Nurses in the M. A. B.', British Journal of Nursing, 11 April 1914, pp. 324-5.

45. Miss Bodley, 'State Aid for Poor Law Nurses', British Journal of Nursing, 13 January 1912, p. 26; Tooley, British

Empire, p. 235; Stansfield, Poor Laws, 1909, p. 504; 'Committee on Workhouse Nursing', Poor Law Officers Journal, 31 January 1902, p. 94.

46.   Miss M. Gardner, 'State Aid as it would affect Nurses', British Journal of Nursing, 25 November 1911, p. 430.

47.   G. Potter, Ministering Angels: The Story of the Royal National Pension Fund for Nurses (The Hospital, London, 1891), p. 25 et seq.

48.   Stansfield, Poor Laws, 1909, p. 504.

49.   Brockbank, M. R. I., p. 62.

50.   W. Whittall, Pensions for Hospital Officers and Staffs, (Layton, London, 1919), p. 29; Brockbank, M. R. I., p. 84.

51.   Whittall, Pensions, p.30.

52.   Stansfield, Poor Laws, 1909, p. 504, p. 614.

53.   Potter, R. N. P. F. N., pp. 57-9.

54.   Mrs. O'Keefe, 'Oral evidence'. See also, Brockbank, M. R. I., p. 101; Strachey, Careers, pp. 78-9.

55.   Cited in Abel-Smith, Nursing Profession, p. 256. In 1938 there were 78,345 registered nurses, of whom 26,091 were hospital nurses and 15,051 were private nurses: the percentage had therefore fallen to approximately 37% in the intervening 25 years. Carter, New Deal, p. 70.

56.   Dr.Bedford Fenwick, Registration of Nurses, 1904, pp. 1-5; M. Breay, 'Nursing in the Victorian Era', Nursing Record and Hospital World, 19 June 1897, pp. 493-502.

57.   'Discussion of Miss Mollett's Paper', British Journal of Nursing, 25 October 1913, p. 333. See also, Tooley, British Empire, p. 278.

58.   Tooley, British Empire, p. 261.

59.   Hospital Records. See also, Maule, 'Training Schools', p. 74; Burdett, Directory, 1898.

60.   Such nurses were warned, however, "that the best class of nurse looks for professional advertisements in a professional paper, and not in a local or county paper." Wilkie, 'Best Means', p. 170.

61.   Howe, Governesses, pp. 125-6; Tooley, British Empire, p. 278.

62.   Banks, Prosperity, p. 205.

63.   Tooley, British Empire, p. 265.

64.   Ibid., p. 265; Burdett, Directory, 1898, p. 431.

65.   Burdett, Directory, 1898. See, however, Vivian, Lectures, p. 95 - "Non-resident posts offer many attractions to Nurses ... but they must remember ... that if, after a while, they wish to return to hospital it will not be very easy to obtain a post. Matrons naturally think they have lost touch with the work and may find it difficult to conform to discipline again." Also footnotes 1 - 3, Chapter 4, above.

66.   Burdett, Succeed, pp. 10-11.

67.   Wilkie, 'Best Means', p. 150.

68.   Stansfield, Poor Laws, 1909, p. 501; White, Social

Change, pp. 95-8, p. 115.

69. Hospital Records; Burdett, Directory, 1898; Burdett, Succeed, p. 75, p. 504; 'My First Workhouse Appointment', Nursing Times, 26 October 1907, p. 936; Davidson, 'Career', p. 58.

70. Mercer, Labour Turnover, p. 149.

71. Ibid., p. 149.

72. Cited in L. Seymer (editor), Selected Writings of Florence Nightingale (MacMillan, New York, 1954), pp. vii-xi, p. 226.

73. H. Swete, Handy Book of Cottage Hospitals (Hamilton Adams, London, 1870), p. 177.

74. Seymer, Selected Writings, p. 227.

75. Strachey, Careers, Preface, np.; Oram, 'Employment'; Tropp, School Teachers, Chapter 1.

76. Tropp, School Teachers, p. 23. Some nurses were uneasy about this exodus; for example, one ex-nurse asked "Why not married Matrons? ... I wonder if the natural and healthy state of holy matrimony would make Matrons as a class more liberal minded?" Cosmopolitan, 'Married Matrons', British Journal of Nursing, 22 May 1909, p. 423.

77. Stansfield, Poor Laws, 1909, p. 613; Mercer, Labour Turnover, p. 11.

78. Miss Luckes, 'Matron's Annual Letter', 1913, The London Hospital, unpublished, p. 41.

79. Terton, Lights and Shadows, p. 71, pp. 84-5.

80. For example, M. E. Loane, An Englishman's Castle (Arnold, London, 1909); A. H. Stoney, In the Days of Queen Victoria (Wright, London, 1910).

81. Seymer, Nightingale's Nurses, p. 19, pp. 44-7, pp. 119-20, p. 152; Carter, New Deal, p. 47.

82. 'First Appointment', pp. 936-7. See also, Smith, People's Health, pp. 388-9; Landale, 'Workhouse Infirmary', p. 7.

83. Landale, 'Workhouse Infirmary', p. 8.

84. 'First Appointment', p. 937.

85. Ibid., p. 937.

86. Landale, 'Workhouse Infirmary', p. 8.

87. Wilkie, 'Best Means', pp. 150-1; Landale, 'Workhouse Infirmary', p. 8; 'Conference', pp. 356-7; E. C. Barton, The History and Progress of Poor Law Nursing (Law and Local Government Publications, London, 1926), p. 8; Stansfield, Poor Laws, 1909, p. 455; Smith, People's Health, p. 368.

88. 'First Appointment', pp. 936-7.

89. Landale, 'Workhouse Infirmary', p. 8.

90. Ibid., p. 8.

91. Stansfield, Poor Laws, 1909, p. 501; S. and B. Webb, State, Chapters 2 - 3; H. Todd, 'Nursing in Poor Law Institutions in England and Wales' in Science and Art of Nursing, pp. 141-2; H. Todd, 'The Report of the Royal Commission on the Poor Laws: V Medical Relief: Indoors', British Journal of

Nursing, 27 March 1909, p. 254; J. F. Oakeshott, 'The Humaniz-
ing of the Poor Law', Fabian Tract, 54, 1894, p. 15.
    92. Hughes, 'Vocation', pp. 101-2.
    93. Landale, 'Workhouse Infirmary', p. 8; L. Dock, 'The
Eugenics Education Society of England', American Journal of
Nursing, August 1905, p. 185.
    94. Burdett, Succeed, p. 8; L. Dock, 'The Status of the
Nurse in the Working World', British Journal of Nursing, 3
January 1914, p. 5.
    95. Dock, 'Status', p. 5. See also Dock, 'Eugenics',
p. 188; Davidson, 'Foundation of Medicine', p. 259; Burdett,
Succeed, p. 17. Tooley wrote that "the district nurse is
something more than a professional worker, she has become a
great factor in social reform. She touches the life of the
poor at every point, and her influence on the homes and on the
habits of the people is almost as important as her care for
the sick." S. Tooley, 'Nursing Past and Present', in Science
and Art of Nursing, p. 22. See also, Tooley, British Empire,
p. 347, p. 352. For a general introduction to the theme of
social imperialism see, G. Lichtheim, Imperialism (Penguin,
London, 1974), p. 16; G. H. Nadel and P. Curtis, Imperialism
(MacMillan, New York, 1964), p. 1; H. Lulty, 'The Passing of
the European Order', Encounter, IX, No. 5, November 1957; B.
Semmel, Imperialism and Social Reform (Allen and Unwin, London,
1960), Chapters 1 and 2; G. R. Searle, The Quest for National
Efficiency (Blackwell, Oxford, 1971); H. C. G. Mathew, The
Liberal Imperialists (O.U.P., London, 1973).

Chapter 5

THE THIRD SEX: SUMMARY AND CONCLUSIONS

> She has a celibate brain but her body is built for delight.[1]

Introduction
No matter how tenuous their links with its reform, commentators were agreed that the evolution of the new nursing order and of its representative, the general trained nurse, was desirable in the interests of the patient and in the furtherance of the science of medicine. The new nurse was 'better' than those she set out to replace, better by virtue of her training and her moral character. By any contemporary criteria, whether it was in-patient mortality rates, bed-occupancy rates or cost-effective hospital management, the general hospitals and their nurses were seen as a significant, if not revolutionary, advance on their predecessors.

So great had the advances in creating high standards of hospital care been that many commentators, including Sidney and Beatrice Webb, argued for the extension of those standards into the domicillary treatment sector. Pointing out that the majority of homes visited by the Poor Law doctors were so filthy and poverty-ridden as to inhibit them from performing their duties, the Webbs recommended that as a minimum nurses were needed to "go before the district medical officer into the miserable home, wash the patient, where practicable change the linen, and by organising the removal of some of the dirt, and generally cleaning up the place, render it possible for him to make a useful diagnosis".[2]

Individually and collectively, the new general nurses were assured of their status and of their distinction not only from other contemporary nurses but from those they superceded. Those who transgressed during training suffered punishment in the form of loss of time or money; those who continued to make mistakes or to flout the code of hospital discipline were castigated as moral delinquents, character failures, and likened to the old nurses of the age of the gamps. The new nurse was aware of her personal evolution through the training programme; she was also aware that she was a privileged member of a new system of nursing which had itself developed out of the dark ages before Nightingale.

In this final chapter we shall take a different approach
to the study of nursing in order to allow us to see more
clearly that evolutionary process at work. By tracing the pro-
genitors of the new nurses through their portrayal in popular
fiction we shall be able to see just how different the new
nurse was, or was expected to be.

Nurses, ladies and skill

With the merest touch of irony and a hint of pathos, Mrs.
Bedford Fenwick recorded, in the Journal she now owned and
edited, the ending of the lady-pupil system of entry to general nursing -

> The Nursing Department at the Middlesex Hospital is
> being modernised, and alas! away go the time honou-
> red L. P.s (lady pupils). These privileged persons
> have long out-lived their raison d'etre ... having
> reformed their system they had no further use for
> her - but in woollen gown and purple ribbons she lin-
> gered long at Middlesex. We need drop no tear at her
> departure, but let us remember with gratitude her use-
> fulness in the past.[3]

Those women who had paid for the privilege of training in
the voluntary hospitals, thereby assuring themselves of hastened promotion to senior posts and of being excused the need
to do 'menial' work whilst training, had, in the early years
of general nursing, played an important role in raising the
moral and class tone of the occupation. They were always few
in number, but if we may read between the lines, were probably
more trouble to the hospitals than they were worth in terms of
income.

As we have noted, the need to train the woman whilst
training the nurse, itself a result of the insufficiency of
middle-class (i.e. lady pupils or paying probationers) entrants to training, put such women out on a limb - they were
already 'ladies' and did not need to be taught how to behave.
Such women usually expected, and nearly always got, separate
accommodation and even separate instruction in the Nurses Home,
considerably increasing the costs of such provisions, and the
isolation of these recruits from the ordinary probationers,
probably hastened their demise. The supernumerary role of the
lady pupil on the wards led to friction, especially as many
apparently saw themselves as "sister's deputies"[4] rather than
as nurses in training: their close social links with the group
from which the doctors were most usually drawn, i.e. the middle-classes, led to problems of relationships between nurses
and doctors on the wards - should a man stand for a lady when
that lady was also a nurse and his professional inferior? In
the end, the lady pupils, having had their day, were phased

out with hardly a note of regret, their place taken now by
the first generation of general hospital trained nurses.

At about the same time as Mrs. Fenwick was recording the
almost unlamented passing of the lady pupil, those general
hospitals offering training were requiring entrants to spend
three years as nurses-in-training; no longer was it possible
for a paying probationer to short-cut the training programme
or for some women to become trained nurses in one or two years.
Even those hospitals which had favoured (usually for financial
reasons rather than training needs), a four-year training had
by and large dropped the fourth year, although some, like the
Western Infirmary, Glasgow, continued to call it a staff-nurse
training year and require its entrants to sign for the full
four years. By 1910 most hospitals offering general training
had adopted a three-year course of instruction, with a series
of examinations at relevant stages in the training programme,
followed by the award of a certificate of competence on completion.

The trained nurse, then, was the skilled nurse: she acquired in each training year specific packages of knowledge
and manual expertise in nursing practices which marked her as
a particular grade of nurse, until she assured her instructors, by passing written and oral examinations, that she had
acquired all those elements of nursing skill which earmarked
the trained general nurse. Nursing skill, then, was defined as
the possession of training and demonstrated by the possession
of a certificate from a 'reputable' hospital: those who called
themselves 'nurse' without these appurtenancies were deceiving
themselves and the public, and were the legitimate objects of
scorn and attack from the real nurses.[5]

We have seen how the trained nurse evolved as a nurse
during her own training and the way in which that training
programme itself had developed, leading to the increasingly
common use of a standard system of nurse training. We may also
demonstrate the way in which the general nurse came to assume
the leadership of the occupation by looking at the sort of
women and nurses she replaced. We know that such women and
nurses were aware of the process we have described as occupational imperialism by the way in which many sought general
nurse training in order to compete with the new nurses, which
in turn reinforced the rhetoric of the process. It may be that
the activities of such 'untrained' nurses also contributed to
their downfall when an alternative became available after the
new nurses emerged from their training hospitals: an examination of those activities may enable us to answer that question.

Nurses and fiction
While we know a good deal about the activities of general
nurses, we know little about the many other types of nurses in
contemporary society. In itself, this would appear to have
been part of the process by which the general nurse sought to

lead the profession, by describing nursing development in terms of the developments only within general nursing; it is also due to the ease of access to data about nursing. Carpenter has begun a study of the mental nurse as "one chapter in the history of labour",[6] and there are a few local studies of district nursing services which fill some of the gaps in our knowledge.[7] However, the non-institutional nurse is almost an unknown quantity in the literature and since many of them would have worked as private nurses on their own account, few have left any records for the historian.

Given the lack of data about non-general nurses and non-institutional nurses in particular, we have to make use of alternative sources of information for any study of the activities of such nurses. A major source for that study is contemporary fiction, novels in which the nurse appears as a character or even as a heroine, and whose actions are essential to the plot or sub-plot, or whose presence in the story allows the author to make some remarks about contemporary attitudes to women and women's work.[8]

In this section of the present study we shall be looking at nursing through the eyes of the novelist and occasionally through the eyes of the reforming novelist, authors such as Charles Reade, Charles Dickens or Elizabeth Gaskell. We should not expect, therefore, bare details of nursing life or mere reportage of nursing events;[9] the material we shall be using forms part of the writer's imagination, and part of the imagination of the reader. Descriptions of nursing practices and of nurses themselves will be bound by the "candy-floss world" of popular fiction,[10] but as long as we are concerned not with the facts within the novel but with attitudes, then the popular fiction of a given period may provide us with valuable insights into contemporary concerns and preoccupations.[11] Fiction of an age can, as Raymond Williams has pointed out, illustrate the "common assumptions" of a class or group, towards a perceived social 'problem' such as industrialisation or the changing role of women in society.[12]

Dependency and exploitation

Perhaps the universal concern to be found in the novel as it discusses the nurse and nursing is the acceptance by the authors of the notion that illness creates dependency, and as a corollary invites exploitation. The care of the sick puts the care-giver in some role which is open to abuse; it is a power relationship which if, as we shall discuss, it goes outside of the immediate family members, and thus involves strangers and hence paid workers, exceeds the 'normal' power relationships which exist within the family.[13]

Florence Nightingale had been aware of the role which family members play in the care of the sick, even writing a nursing vade mecum for those who looked after ill relations;[14] however, she, like her contemporaries, saw such care-givers as

148

female relatives since the natural role for women included the caring through health and through sickness of the woman's own family as mother, wife, daughter and sister. Nightingale's recognition of the dependency of the ill person and the potential exploitation of them by female relatives led her to remind her readers of their natural functions as care-givers -

> Almost every woman in England has, at one time or
> another of her life, charge of the personal health
> of somebody, whether child or invalid ... If, then,
> every woman must, at some time or another in her
> life become a nurse ... how immense and how valu-
> able it would be if every woman would think how to
> nurse. (original emphasis).[15]

- a reminder not only of their innate abilities and duties but of their responsibilies not to exceed their position of trust.

In Nightingale's own work responses to dependency in the sickroom and the potential for exploitation were translated into the need and obligation to make the sick person comfortable and clean, and included creeping about silently rather than crashing about with little regard to the heightened sensitivity of the sick person, as well as following precisely the doctor's orders rather than any intuitive or wise-woman methods of caring. These learnt skills and knowledge, she went on to argue, were the proper sphere not of the untrained female relative, no matter how dutiful she might be, but of the trained nurse alone.[16]

Nurses and the novels
It is a remarkable coincidence that the first novel in which nursing and nurses appear as subjects for comment was also one of the first examples of the form of fiction which we recognise as a novel. The Journal of the Plague Year (1722) written by Daniel Defoe had as one of its objects the attempt to mingle "fact with fiction" and to "treat fiction as fact", in order to better present the author's attack on contemporary mismanagement of the apparatus of State, exemplified by its inability to protect the middle-classes during the outbreak of plague in London in 1665, and its inability to provide humanitarian care for the poor during that awful catastrophe.

The nurses in that work are hardly characters, nor even the caricatures they appear in Dickens' Martin Chuzzlewit (1843/44), but in a novel in which there is hardly a recognisable plot and certainly no hero, that is not too surprising. The development of the nurse as a character and eventually as a heroine took over 150 years, and when she did appear as a heroine in her own right she was, significantly enough, a general hospital nurse. Nurse Elisia (1893) tells us little about the standards of in-patient care in the wards of a London voluntary hospital but a considerable amount about the

transition and resulting conflict from every-woman-as-nurse to
trained woman-as-nurse. Rather than look in detail at each of
our selected novels in which the nurse or her work is discussed, we shall attempt to identify the way in which the contemporary concerns about nurses and nursing are presented and
change over time, as developments in the wider world influence
authors' perceptions and readers' imaginations.

For Defoe the dependency of sickness and its expolitation
were far more real and invidious than it had been even for
Nightingale. His nurses, the "hired nurses" who looked after
the plague victims, used their positions of trust to cheat
and steal from their clients, even to murder them; there were,
he wrote in his <u>Journal</u> ... ,

> vast numbers that went about as nurses to tend those
> that were sick, they committed a great many thieve-
> ries in the houses where they were employed; and
> some of them were publicly whipped for it, when per-
> haps they ought rather to have been hanged for exam-
> ples, for numbers of houses were robbed on these oc-
> casions, till at length the parish officers were
> sent to recommend nurses to the sick, and always
> took account of whom it was they sent, so as they
> might call them to account if the house had been ab-
> used where they had been placed ...
>   They did tell me, indeed, of a nurse in one
> place that laid a wet cloth upon the face of a dying
> patient who she tended and so put an end to his life,
> who was expiring just before; and another that smo-
> thered a young woman she was looking to when she was
> in a fainting fit, and would have come to herself;
> some that killed them by giving them one thing, some
> another, and some starved them by giving nothing at
> all.[17]

The stories about the nurses mistreating and even murder-
ing their patients forced many of those who needed their services to shun them - "they grew more cautious whom they took
into their houses, and whom they trusted their lives with, and
had them always recommended if they could" - but for those who
could find no such reliable nurses i.e. the poorest classes,
"the misery of that time lay upon (them)". Such victims were
unable to find a doctor, apothecary or nurse to attend to them
and thus they "died calling for help".[18]
Even though the novelist admitted that there was "more of
tale than of truth" in his story, (a common literary device),
the sense of incapacity in the face of disease ran over into
Defoe's proffered means of overcoming such catastrophes. For
Defoe illness, especially an epidemic, was divinely-inspired
and could only be relieved or overcome by recourse to God and
His works.[19] Defoe's alternative nurse was, therefore, the

good christian woman, the good wife; not only did she care
for her own family but because of her christian charity she
also went out and cared for the poor who were friendless and
without family. Mrs. John Hayward "tended many that died in
the parish being for her honesty recommended by the parish
officers", and rather than reaping the material but transi-
tory and often ill-gotten rewards in this life, she, and
others like her, received public recognition of her virtue
and divine acknowledgement of her works, since "she was never
infected" by the plague.[20]

The perils of sickness could force even the members of
the ruling classes into dependent roles, as had happened to
the uncle of the hero of Richardson's second novel, The History of Sir Charles Grandison (1754). In that work, the nurse
had been employed to help Lord W. recover from some illness
but had gone beyond the sick-nurse role by becoming the mistress and housekeeper of the earl. Mrs. Giffard, the nurse,
and Lord W. had entered into this carnal relationship with
open eyes and with proper legal provision made for either
party wishing to break the relationship. A settlement was
agreed on, to be paid to the nurse if and when she left, but
in the plot she is seen abusing her close physical and emotional ties with the earl to demand an increased allowance
which the earl, in his dependent and exploited role, cannot
but agree to. The honour of the family and the purse of Lord
W. are saved by the appearance of the hero, the Sir Charles
of the title, who offers the nurse a bribe to encourage her
to leave without too much fuss.

While Richardson was probably more concerned with contemporary morals amongst the ruling classes rather than nurses
per se, his depiction of the nurse as a person who can use
the dependency of the ill-person for pecuniary advantage via
sexuality reflected the view that such occurences, while not
necessarily common, were possible. The nurse, of course, plays
a similar role in The History ... as did the domestic servant
in Richardson's earlier novel, Pamela (1741): either could
use their privileged and peculiar position within the household to defraud the employer or to lead an employer into unacceptable moral situations.

The nurse as sexual vampire is a recurring theme throughout the period, and, indeed, beyond;[21] either a patient is be-
witched, as happened to Lord W., or else, and in particular
towards the end of the nineteenth-century, she distracted the
hero - usually a young doctor - from his obvious path towards
a career and good marriage. This latter role for the nurse
may be seen in any of the novels written after the 1890's,
when the new nurses had emerged from their training schools
to be recognised as potential competitors to the doctors who
were at the same time establishing and asserting their professional status. As an illustration we might profitably look
in detail at Trelawney's novel, In a Cottage Hospital (1901),

set in the fictional country town of Rebley. The hero of the
novel is Dr. Kargill, a newly qualified doctor, whose appointment to Rebley cottage hospital is to be the prelude to a promising surgical career, probably as a London consultant. The
heroine is Nurse May Patterson, a "perfect woman" in Kargill's
eyes, but who appears to be only an average nurse on duty.

May was a "pleasant, smiling girl with a mass of fair
wavy hair", who strikes Kargill the doctor as "the most fas-
cinating woman he had ever met": in part, of course, this is
because he has not met many others since, like all socially
mobile entrants to the professions, his studies had taken up
all of his time. But the fascination for May has another aspect; May awakens in him a "desparate sexual longing" and it
is this which almost brings about Kargill's disgrace.

Rebley, like the entire cottage hospital system Trelawney
thought needed reform,[22] is badly and corruptly managed, the
vice extending downwards from the "consultants" through the
lay administrator and the matron to the nurses themselves. At
the root of the corruption, however, is sex or its bourgeois
equivalent, money: the consultants have affairs with the nurses and perform illegal abortions; the administrator accepts
bribes for supplies contracts, and the matron allows room for
the nurses to liaise with the doctors by being herself sexually
involved with an itinerant bogus preacher.

Kargill, fresh from medical school, realises that the
poor standard of care is intolerable and determines to reform
the hospital; in this task he almost succeeds until he is discovered in the arms of the dying May. She had had an abortion,
performed by one of Rebley's 'consultants', Kargill's superior
and enemy. The hero's attempts to reform the hospital begin to
fall away as he appears to be one of the corrupt himself, a
situation he is rescued from only by the timely arrival of a
detective who investigates May's death and shows Kargill to be
blameless and the consultant the guilty party.

The reforms then go on apace, but too late for Kargill;
his love and the cause of his partial disgrace is now dead and
he leaves the hospital for the war in South Africa, only to be
posted missing soon after his arrival there. May the nurse,
who was not a good nurse since she could not be trusted to
carry out Kargill's professional instructions, and May the
woman are the cause of the young doctor's failure; sex and
professional incompetence are not too far apart; the inexperienced lover, Kargill, is diverted (almost) from his professional duty and it takes the death of the experienced partner
in the affair, the nurse, to allow reforms to take place.

The nurse as sexual spider to the inexperienced or easily
impressed young doctor, was a common theme in many romance
novels, for example G. M. Fenn's Nurse Elisia (1893); Mrs.
Haycraft's Sister Royal (c1900) and J. J. Abraham's The Night
Nurse (1913). It was such a common literary device that, in
The Night Nurse, Abraham had one of his minor characters re-

hearse the discussion about the problems of young male doctors working alongside young female nurses. The doctor, according to this consultant-character, had to develop a special relationship with the nurse; he had to overcome - as quickly as possible for his career's sake - the "nurse-fever stage" and come to regard the nurse in a special, asexual way.[23]

Nowhere was the dependency of the ill-person and the exploitative nature of the nurse-role so well exposed as in Charles Dickens' novel <u>Martin Chuzzlewit</u>. While the characters of Sarah Gamp and Betsy Prig are more caricatures than players, even in a sub-plot, the attitudes felt by some sections of society, in particular the lower middle-classes and petit-bourgeoisie which had thrown up Dickens himself, to the dangers of falling ill in the changed society of Victorian England are ably and alarmingly described.[24]

In the Preface to the 1868 edition of the novel, Dickens had insisted that Mrs. Gamp and Mrs. Prig were "fair representations" of contemporary private and hospital nurses. In an oft-quoted passage from the sub-plot, a hapless and friendless patient, who is suffering from an unspecified fever, is "bad abed" and Sarah and Betsy have been engaged to tend him. The young man was lying almost motionless in the bed, except that his head was continuously rolling from side to side on the pillow, a sight which caused Sarah some distress only solaced by a liberal pinch of snuff. Having made sure that she would be comfortable during the long night and having assured herself of her escape in the event of a fire, Sarah gave the slime draught to the patient by "the simple process of clutching the patient's windpipe to make him gasp, and immediately pouring it down his throat". She then turned herself into a "watcher of the sick", that is, a nurse, by making herself a bed, dressing herself as for retiring and lighting a rushlight candle. The night-long ramblings of the fevered patient not only bring forth repartee from the nurse but timely opportunities for her to refresh herself with her supper: occasionally the ramblings call forth threats of physical violence from Sarah, since they interrupt her sleep, but no actual assault takes place.

Against this total lack of humanity the patient has no redress; it is unfortunate he is ill and it is his bad luck to be far from home and friends, at the mercy of strangers who will not care for him in the way his family could be expected to. But was Dickens correct in this assertion, would the patient have fared any better in the bosom of his family? According to some novelists, who were at pains to show what modern nursing was like and how it was allied to scientific medicine and required a proper training, he would not.

In Charlotte Bronte's <u>Shirley</u> (1849) the female relatives of the hero rally round and nurse him when he is injured in a riot, but they turn out to be an impediment to his recovery. The surgeon, MacTurk, had diagnosed a life-threatening condi-

tion and had suggested the family should employ a nurse he
would recommend: this the family would not do and the female
relatives, Mrs. Yorke and Hortense, "promised faithfully observation of directions. He was left, therefore, for the present in their hands. Doubtless, they executed the trust to the
best of their ability: but something got wrong: the bandages
were displaced or tampered with: great loss of blood followed.
MacTurk being summoned, came with great stead afoam", - and
after a few coarse epithets against "meddling womanhood", the
surgeon had his way and brought in a trained nurse. With the
care of the nurse, Zillah Horsfall, and the skill of the surgeon, the hero recovered speedily; it is unclear whether the
pace of the recovery was due to the high standard of care
given by the nurse or as a direct result of her physically
repulsive demeanour and manners.

Even the aristocratic hospital nurse, Nurse Elisia in the
novel of that name, who had none of the coarseness of Mrs.
Horsfall, found it difficult to overcome the resentment of the
female relatives at their exclusion from their natural sphere,
the sickroom. The elderly aunt of the hero's father in Fenn's
novel fears that the unknown nurse coming to look after her
brother who has had a stroke after a riding accident will not
be trustworthy; her experience of nurses is "that they are
dreadful women, who drink and go to sleep in the sickrooms,
and the patients cannot wake them and dies for want of attention". The dependency of the sickroom and the exploitation by
the nurse were the real fears of the class employing such
nurses 'sight unseen', and even the local labouring-classes
feel that it is a mistake to trust such outsiders.[25] It takes
the intervention of the youngest female relative to help the
new nurse integrate her role within the private domain, where
by her skill and patience her status becomes established and
accepted.

Nursing and work in the novel

It would appear, then, that as the nurse characterisation developed, the fears about exploitation through sickness were
translated from absolute immorality into the usurping of
natural roles, particularly for female relatives. It is surely
no mere coincidence that Nightingale and other nurse-reformers
were discussing the way in which women needed training in
order to nurse more effectively at the same time as novelists
were posing in their own way the debate over women's natural
sphere; nor that both were going on at the same time as many
more contemporaries were concerning themselves with the problem of the surplus women of the middle classes.

We may see the way in which some commentators saw a solu-
tion to that surplus in the opening up of new work opportunities for women through our discussion of nursing in the popular novels of the period. For example, as we have noted, there
was a need, if nursing was to become suitable as paid work for

such women - and not just as another area of charitable endea-
vour - for it to be reformed, or at least taken out of the
hands of the incumbents - mainly working-class married women.
Nursing had to become an acquired skill, a profession, since
by making it so it would be possible to exclude some women who
were considered unsuitable: nursing could not belong to every-
woman, but only to some women. Those women were to be trained
nurses and eventually, as we have discussed, trained nurses
and trained women. In the early years, however, it was training which was emphasised and, since training required expenditure, it was only available to those who could afford it,
either because they already had sufficient income not to need
to work for wages, or else they were willing to forgo earning
reasonable wages until they had acquired the attributes of a
trained nurse: nurses of the modern period were to be either
paying pupils, lady-pupils, or probationers in training.

Contemporary fascination with the plight of the surplus
woman meshed with a fascination with why women would willingly
work amid sickness and disease. In Rosa M. Carey's novel
Merle's Crusade (1889) the heroine, Merle, is one of the surplus women, parentless and taken in by her aunt and uncle until she is out of her teens, when she comes to realise that
she is a financial burden to them, no matter how much they
love her. While Anthony Trollope had argued that the only
suitable career for a woman was marriage,[26] Merle could point
out to her uncle when he echoed Trollope's sentiments that for
girls like her marriage was a declining possibility -

> Women are crying out for work, Uncle Keith, I con-
> tinued, carrying my warfare into a fresh quarter ...
> There are too many of the poor things in this
> world, and the female market is overstocked ... [27]

Nursing appeared as the quintescence of motherhood to
those whose chances of becoming biological mothers was remote,
like Merle and her sisters-in-kind: "to serve others seems the
very meaning of womanhood; in some sense a woman serves all
the days of her life", and she might as well do that as a
trained nurse.[28]

Motive for nursing, then, was tied up with chances of
marriage, at least in the popular fiction; even those women
who could have married but appear to choose to nurse instead
posed little problem for the author since, in keeping with the
happy-ending genre, these women find themselves married in the
closing passages of the novels.[29] But it was recognised that
some women might choose to nurse rather than take up the offer
of marriage; Nightingale has been portrayed in this way, although there is no evidence to suggest that she substituted
nursing for marriage on return from the Crimea, since she
hardly nursed afterwards. Her reforming zeal in nursing and
in other affairs was quite within the compass of a married

woman as many campaigns found to their benefit in the period. Novelists remained fascinated, however, with this apparent choice to nurse, whether it was related to chances of marriage or not.

Defoe argued that women turned to nursing, especially nursing the dying, in order to get material reward from their work; nursing, or at least paid nursing, was not a vocation or a calling. In the eighteenth-century, then, only the philanthropic Mrs. Hayward and her ilk were true nurses because they were true women; accepting payment for nursing duties, no matter how much individuals might need an income, almost certainly would result in the debasement of the woman by exposing her to the devil's work, sickness, a temptation she would be unable to resist having taken the first and fatal step to accept payment for her christian duty.

Sarah Gamp was a widow who was forced to nurse to support herself, and the need for income had led to her debasement; in Elisabeth Gaskell's novel Ruth (1853), the heroine turns to nursing not to earn a living, and thus place herself in the potentially damning position on the road to gampism, but as a means of attonement for a previous sin. Ruth, through her own fault since she had known what she was doing, was made pregnant by her lover who then deserts her. After the child's birth Ruth finds herself an outcast and eventually is taken into the household of a dissenting minister and his sister. There she stays, and in order not to be a burden to them, Ruth works as a daily governess and passes herself off as a widow. When a typhoid epidemic strikes the town, and all are afraid to help in the local fever hospital, Ruth volunteers her services because her lies have been discovered. Her work with the sufferers, she believes, will almost certainly end in her own death which she feels will atone for her previous bad life. By a twist of fate or irony she survives the epidemic but succumbs to it when she nurses her ex-lover later; Ruth dies and her sin with her.

While Nightingale was apparently pleased that Ruth had had some experience of nursing in an institution - the fever hospital - before nursing a private case - her ex-lover -, and apparently found the novel enjoyable,[30] Ruth's motives for nursing may have caused her some anxiety in her reforming mission. Nightingale did not want for her new nurses women who had had "a disappointment in love, the want of an object, a general disgust, or incapacity for other things".[31] On those grounds she would have rejected not only Ruth but also Marcella, the heroine of Mrs. Humphrey Ward's novel (1894). Marcella was the daughter of a petty aristocrat who spent some time in her late teens and early womanhood in London, studying art among the bohemian set where she also learnt at first hand of the distress amongst the lower orders. A bitter row between a potential suitor and Marcella sends her off to do some good, especially since the row had been actuated by the suffering she had witnessed on her father's estate. Back in London she trains as a nurse in a voluntary hospital before taking up a post with a charitable district nursing organisation, working in the slums of the metropolis.

In that novel the familiar concerns and even scorn for those who took up work instead of marriage (since it brought reality uncomfortably close for many others) is shown by the attitudes of Marcella's social peers, one of whom, Lady Selina, thought that nursing was "all that the women do nowadays, they tell me, who can't get on with their relations or their lovers".[32] Some of these contemporaries also suspected that these nurse entrants would not really experience the full horrors of the work, protected by their money and their social class. However, a more direct criticism of such wealthy and philanthropic ladies entering nursing was not that they themselves were misdirected but that they were not being the most effective in their charity. If such women were really concerned about the plight of the poorer classes then they should really think carefully about how best to remedy their lot. Nursing, they argued, may be "magnificant" but it really was "hardly business from her point of view. How much more she might have done for the poor with thirty thousand a year". In other words, individual self-sacrifice was wasteful of the inherent talents of the elite class; they should keep out of the actual work itself and instead organise others to do it and do it efficiently.

The first example we have of a woman who sees in nursing not escape from an unhappy love affair or restrictive parents, or a means of redressing a personal wrong or a humanitarian concern which is misguided, but who sees in nursing work as a means of self-fulfillment is in Abraham's novel The Night Nurse (1913). The heroine, Nora, chooses to work and to reject marriage not because she is unhappy or especially socially concerned but because she believes that she can achieve her potential as a human being through work, just as men do. Nora is not one of the redundant women with little chance of marriage nor has she sinned; Nora Townsend is the first new nurse who is also a "New Woman".[33] For her "getting married has no attractions"; "most women seem to marry for a home. I used to think that degrading till I came to see it was largely due to their economic dependence". Since she has found work which makes her independent she does not need a home, and hence a husband, and "all this talk about love leaves (her) cold".[34]

Nora is not an old maid, but a "batchelor woman",[35] a woman who "is beginning to find out that she, not man, is the race; that she can carry on the work of that race almost completely without him; and that there are not too many women in the world but too many men."[36] For her nursing is part of her self-fulfillment and marriage is not an issue. Naturally the novelist, having allowed his characters full range for their new ideas, including those about the future of the race and

the eugenics movement, brings the hero and heroine together to
make a happy ending, thus comforting his readers without un-
duly upsetting his characterisations, since in the end it is
they, as members of the elite, who ought to marry and produce
the future race.[37]

The fascination with the type of woman who nursed and why
she did so continued to find expression in the novel through
the work of the nurse and the helplessness of the sick person.
Defoe had written about the nursing of the dying and the lay-
ing-out of the dead, tasks which Sarah Gamp frequently performed. Unlike Defoe's nurses, however, Dickens' characters
also nursed cases likely to recover, or at least who ought to
have recovered. His nurses gave out medicines, as we noted,
and watched the patient - a procedure which was designed not
merely to observe the the fight between life and death in the
human frame but to obtain an accurate record of that struggle
so that it might be reported to the doctor, who would then
adapt his heroic intervention if necessary. Of course,
Dickens' nurses failed to carry out this elementary task, just
as they failed to administer medicines in a humane way; the
doctor is, therefore, little the wiser for their report -

> The doctor came too, the doctor shook his head. It
> was all he could do, under the circumstances, and
> he did it well.
> What sort of a night, nurse?
> Restless, sir, said Mrs. Gamp
> Talk much?
> Middling, sir, said Mrs. Gamp.
> Nothing to the purpose, I suppose?
> Oh, bless you, no, sir. Only jargon.
> Well, said the doctor, we must keep him quiet;
> keep his draughts regularly; and see that he's
> carefully looked to. That's all.
> And as long as Mrs. Prig and me waits upon him, sir,
> no fear of that; said Mrs. Gamp.[38]

Apart from the slime draught, Sarah's patient is hardly
bothered by the nurse who does little for him except watch
and curse him for disturbing her; Nurse Elisia, the aristo-
crat-nurse, however, does do something to relieve the suffering of her patients, but it is only described as relieving the
sufferer by rubbing eau-de-cologne on a patient's brow. Even
Marcella, who on the district finds a bad case of puerperal
fever, is shown only vaguely doing things, although her reporting, unlike Sarah's, is much better organised and even
charted.[39]

As we noted earlier, we should not look in the novel for
the "rare details"[40] of the nurses' work but rather for changing attitudes to nurses and nursing. We have so far noted how
paid nursing was seen as debasing and was replaced by philan-

158

thropic enterprise, which in turn was replaced by a return to paid but now trained nursing: we have also noted that the fear of illness and the dependency which it engendered caused many novelists to examine the relationships between nurse and patient, and between nurse and woman.

That fear, whether rational or not, did not only apply to physical illness and its dependency; indeed, it was mental illness and incarceration in an asylum for the insane which appears to have been the focus of many apprehensions voiced about the relationship between illness and nursing as well, of course, illness and medicine itself. Charles Reade enjoyed considerable contemporary success as a popular novelist who often used his work to highlight a social problem. In one of his novels, Hard Cash (1863), he set out to expose the current state of the private mad-house system, and the ease with which a minor could be incarcerated against his will and without due medical cause, enabling relatives to defraud him of his inheritance. While Reade might have more profitably exposed the use of asylums as a last recourse of help for many single women, like the governesses said to make up such a proportion of the inmates of asylums,[41] there is in the novel a vivid expose of contemporary mental care and types of treatment then in vogue.[42] Since the novel also describes some of the sorts of women found as nurses in such institutions we may profitably look at some of the details found in this social-conscience novel.

The hero, if he can be so described, of Hard Cash is Alfred, a somewhat slow-witted young man who has been sent to the asylum by his own father, in collusion with a doctor, in order to defraud him of his inheritance. One of the treatments given for mania in the asylum is "tanking", the immersion of the patient in water in order to soothe the passions. However, the treatment had become a punishment, given for the least offence against the regulations of the asylum or of disrespect to the officials,

> or out of mere wantoness, they would drag a pa-
> tient stark naked across the yard, and thrust her
> bodily under the water again and again, keeping
> her down until almost gone with suffocation, and
> dismissing her more dead than alive with obscene
> and insulting comments ringing in her ears, to
> get warm in the cold.[43]

The treatment, when properly carried out, i.e. on medical orders, was given during the morning ablutions but "without suffocating" the patient; however, the total immersion of the body in cold water, when accepted medical opinion recommended warm water, "was a severe trial to those numerous patients in whom the circulation was weak". When used as a punishment or for the sadistic pleasure of a 'nurse' or "keeperess", up to

twenty patients at a time would be tanked and then they would
be served the "foul water for their meals". Even a pregnant
patient could not avoid the tank if it so pleased the nurses,
and even though one of them objects to it she merely tells the
hero of her feelings without actually stopping the cruelty.[44]

Not only were the treatments in the asylum debased by the
nurses, the nurses themselves were debased examples of the
group they represent. The nurse who has most day to day contact with the hero, Nurse Hannah, and whom he hopes to enlist
in his bid to be released, is shown to be a mongrel version of
womanhood:

> presently Nurse Hannah came bustling along with an
> apronful of things, and let herself into a vacant
> room hard by. This Hannah was a young women with a
> pretty and rather babyish face, diversified by a
> thick biceps muscle in her arm that a blacksmith
> need not have blushed for. And I suspect it was
> this masculine charm, and not her feminine fea-
> tures that had won her the confidence of Baker &
> Co., and the respect of her female patients: big
> or little, excited or not, there was not one of
> them this bicipital baby-face could not pin by the
> wrists, and twist her helpless into a strong-room,
> or handcuff her unaided in a moment; and she did
> too, on slight provocation.[45]

The work of an asylum nurse, Reade argued, could lead any
feminine woman to develop the harshness of the masculine character, turn her into a "Baby-faced Biceps", especially if the
institution was mismanaged because it served a purpose other
than that of caring for the deranged in an humane way. Such
sentiments, as we have seen, were reflections of a general anxiety about the affects of nursing, and other work, on femininity.

Nurses and doctors
One of Dickens' side-swipes in his attack on contemporary nursing was a criticism of the state of medicine itself: remember
that he had written that "the doctor shook his head. It was
all he could do under the circumstances, and he did it well".
This concern was not only about doctors, per se, a common
theme in many novels,[46] but was as much a statement about the
relationship between the male doctor and the female nurse,
which in Dickens' work was presented as a demand for the close
supervision of nurses by good doctors.

In Bronte's novel, Shirley, the nurse, Mrs. Horsfall, is
brought in by the doctor and was "the best nurse on his staff".
While she drinks and smokes like Sarah Gamp, she is completely
trustworthy as far as her technical competence is concerned.
Having been trained by MacTurk she has the prime virtue that

"drunk or sober, she always remembers to obey" the doctor. The absolute loyalty demanded of a nurse by a doctor is shown in the character of Zillah Horsfall and her behaviour towards the patient and his relatives, whom she immediately excludes from the sickroom. MacTurk regarded himself as a mechanic and his patients as damaged machinery and required that his nurse have the same attitudes; Mrs. Horsfall was a mechanical extension of the surgeon's arm, a robot for the repair of the human frame.[47]

Nurse Elisia's relationships with doctors was easier and more 'human' in regard to care but complicated by her class relationships with medical men; Marcella had the same sort of class difficulties, but being a properly trained general hospital nurse, class was unimportant as long as nursing skill was needed and paramount. Marcella's greatest difficulty with doctors came when she suspects one of them of mistreating her patient, when she also suspects him of a class prejudice against the poor whom she is nursing.

In a graphic account of the conditions faced by many nurses working in the slums of inner London, Mrs. Ward describes Marcella at work with a woman suffering from puerperal fever. It was "what a nurse calls a 'good case', one that rouses all her nursing skills and faculty", and throughout a long night the nurse battles bravely - although without any real detail we cannot know how the battle was fought - to pull the young mother through. In the morning she prepares herself and her patient for the arrival of the doctor - by sweeping and cleaning and other tasks which the Webbs were to later recommend the nurse of the poor to do[48] - and by compiling her case notes and charts for his inspection.[49]

When the doctor arrives, Marcella is disturbed by the patient's shrinking away from his touch and begins to suspect him of a degree of callousness which she thinks he would not have in the presence of a lady.[50] When he disregards her observations - scientific nursing observations - and when she smells brandy on his breath, she decides that her patient should not be exposed to further risk of neglect. She confronts the doctor and tells him to go, leave the patient to her care: in the face of such a direct challenge to his authority the doctor explodes, almost to the point of striking the nurse. Asked if she knows her place, Marcella faces up to this onslaught by reminding the doctor that she is a trained nurse of the new order; answering him with a definite "Yes, I know my place", she shows that she is aware of the proper relationships between nurse and doctor. Marcella knew from her own skill and knowledge of medicine that the doctor had endangered the patient's life by his neglect and that "he was in a fair way to endanger it again" and this, together with the courage born of her humanitarian principles, allowed her to speak up on behalf of the poor woman.[51]

The doctor, faced with such an attack on his professional

and personal standing has no answer except, almost, violence: he storms off vowing not to treat the patient until another nurse has been assigned to the case. The sort of nurse he wanted was one who will instantly obey his orders without questioning them and without perhaps any real understanding of their significance: in other words, this sort of doctor would "sooner have one old Gamp" than any of the new trained nurses.[52]

The conflict of authority between doctors and nurses was generally defused by the training regime which the new nurses underwent and only surfaced when the doctor or the nurse were of the old system and hence a danger to the new order of medicine or nursing. Changes in the relationships between men and women in society in general had altered so that blind obedience was no longer demanded of a wife, rather a shared common ground of mutual trust and belief, so that conflict could not appear. In nursing that common ground was the professional relationship between the trained nurse and the doctor, where her skill and knowledge enabled the nurse to carry out the instructions of the doctor not with criticism but with understanding and thus without question. If she understood the reasons for the instructions or decisions, she would not question them or the doctor; her training allowed the nurse to have that understanding.

The doctors were also expected to play their part in this process of inter-professional relationships; they were to be involved in nurse training and in explanation and in treating the new nurse as a complementary assistant. As one nursing manual written by a doctor put it, the doctor was the captain of a ship, the nurse the first mate, although that author seems to have forgotten that the possibility existed for a first mate to become a captain; the analogy did, however, spell out the respective spheres for nurses and doctors.[53]

But the doctor was also presumed to be a disciplinary figure in the nursing world; the rituals of behaviour expected of the nurse in his presence were illustrations of that role. By maintaining a distance between nurse and doctor, by a coldness, reserve and lack of familiarity between them, the doctor could exert a moral and disciplinary control over the nurse and her activities. Thus, when Kargill found himself involved emotionally with Nurse May his attempts at doing his job effectively and his attempts to reform the hospital are almost thwarted.

Nurses and authority

There were other authority figures in the nursing world beside the medical men; the three tier system of hospital authority experienced by many today had its origins in the structures of nineteenth-century hospitals, with the medical authority supplemented and enhanced first of all by lay administrators and then by the nurses themselves.

The lack of control over nurses and nursing services for the poor by the lay administrators was criticised in the Journal of the Plague Year, where the local Poor Law authorities had the responsibility for providing proper medical and nursing facilities during the epidemic. The unfortunate sick poor of London found little help forthcoming from the parish officers and only those who made direct appeal to the Lord Mayor gained any relief from their distress; it was only when public outcry had reached a high level that the parish officers eventually accepted their responsibilities in the matter and began to recommend good sick nurses to the poor. Those recommended by the parish officials, because they had legal duties, etc., were often very good as nurses and earned the commendation of the parish officers as well as the thanks of their patients; one such was, of course, Mrs. John Hayward.

At Rebley Cottage Hospital, the lay administration was corrupt with the hospital Secretary accepting bribes to place contracts for goods and services in the hands of relatives and friends in the town. The corruption of the Secretary meant that when Kargill attempted to get some essential equipment which a modern hospital ought to have, he failed since the Secretary had falsified the books to give the impression that it was already available to the doctors.

Overall lack of control over supplies at Rebley extended to the ward stocks, including the medicinal brandy which the nurses drank at one of their supper parties. Since the Matron was aware of the inaccuracies in the hospital supplies system and rather than exposing them actually takes advantage of them herself, the lay control over nursing affairs was bound to be infected with the seeds of corruption. If the head of the nursing staff was implicated in the scandals of maladministration, then it was inevitable, according to the novelist, that the lower ranks should also be affected.

The ward sisters at Rebley were familiar with the nurses, smoking and drinking with them at parties and even found walking arm in arm noisily through the hospital corridors. Such behaviour was not conducive to good nursing discipline and as a direct consequence the standard of care given by the nurses at the cottage hospital was appallingly lax. Kargill found out just how low that standard was when he did his night-rounds and came across a distressed female patient, who called out to him. The night sister tells the patient to be quiet, explaining to the doctor that the woman is only a "stupid girl" "who has had her leg put up in plaster and has been annoying" the nurses ever since. Investigating further Kargill finds

a young girl, certainly not yet out of her teens. Her face exhibited traces of evident suffering and there was a bright red patch on each cheek, which contrasted markedly with the waxy pallor of the rest of her skin. The bed-clothes at the end of

163

the bed were raised over a wire cradle which kept
them from contact with her injured leg. Kargill
felt her pulse. It was abnormally rapid and her
hand was burning hot. He looked at the temperature chart which hung by the side of the bed, but
no observations appeared to have been recorded
upon it since the patient's admission.[54]

It appeared immediately obvious to Kargill that the leg
had been badly set, causing the pain and fever: his surprise
at finding that it had been the Matron herself who had put the
leg into plaster is matched by the discovery that there is no
medicinal brandy on the ward to give to the patient as a
stimulant. He eventually relieves the sufferings of the poor
girl but without the active assistance of the night sister,
who merely stands to one side of the bed, silently mocking
him.

The doctor's fears about the lack of control over nursing
practices by the sisters and, of course, by the other doctors
are confirmed when he later visits a men's ward. There he is
asked to perform duties which the patients should expect the
nurses to do, "the sundry necessaries" such as giving bedpans
and urinals, giving out drinks; when he asks one patient where
the nurse is, the patient admits that he does not know and
that she has not been seen for over an hour. Furthermore, the
patient claims that "yer 'ere to look after yerself in this
bloomin' place at nights". It transpires that the nurses are
off "canoodlin'; aloving up an' kissen fellers as they gets in
ter supper with 'em". The nurses, according to the patients,
"dunna care if yer dies for a drink o'water or bursts yersel
for lack of their hattention".[55]

We can see, in the extreme case of Rebley, the contemporary novelist's concern with the question of control over
nursing which Defoe had originally spelt out in his Journal...
- the need for the nurse to be subject to some higher authority than herself. This could take the form of christian responsibility to one's neighbour and thus God, or could be supplemented by the existence of mortal representations of that
authority, i.e. men, doctors or lay administrators. Since, as
we have noted, the doctor and the lay administrator were increasingly distancing themselves from direct control over
nursing affairs, the nurses themselves had to fill in the gap
left in the authority structure. That gap was filled by the
matron and by the ward sisters, with the hierarchy of nursing
authority eventually added to by the inclusion of the home
sister and the sister tutor figures.

However, because the new trained nurse was also a trained
woman, part of the control over the nurse was vested in the
nurse herself, and we have shown how the training and socialisation of the nurse helped that self-control develop. Self-
control could enable all the elements of authority over nurs-

ing to be directed from a distance; in any situation the nurse could be relied upon to behave because she had been trained to control herself along desired lines. As an aid for the nurse to remember how she exercised self-control, and how she differed from other 'nurses', key elements in the nurse/doctor/administrator relationships were identified and codified, one extreme example being that of the Nightingale Oath.

The Oath was originally a part of the syllabus of training at St. Thomas's Hospital, London, where the nurses were expected to be "Sober, Honest, Truthful, Trustworthy, Punctual, Quiet and Orderly, Cleanly and Neat, Patient, Cheerful and Kindly".[56] Nightingale's own elaboration of these virtues also included "chaste, in the sense of the Sermon on the Mount", as well as detailed interpretations of how each virtue was demonstrated in action.[57]

If we were to extract key concerns about nurses and their actions from contemporary fiction involving nurse characterisations, we should find a close similarity between those fictional concerns and the Nightingale Oath. Sarah Gamp was given to drink as was Zillah Horsfall: Sarah could not be trusted to stay awake and the nurses at Rebley could not be trusted to nurse their patients: Defoe's nurses stole from their dying patients, Sarah Gamp stole time from her duty and the Rebley nurses purloined the brandy intended for the patients.[58]

The new nurses, then, whether fictional or real, were different from their predecessors in almost every respect, but that development did not come automatically, as the plot motifs in the novels show. Contemporary concern about the changing role of women in society, about the professionalisation of medicine and the new occupations for women, are all re-presented in the novels as they concern nurses and nursing. Just as the actual social developments took time to work through, so, too, did the attitudes expressed in fiction take time to develop. While there may be broad similarities between the concerns expressed by Defoe in the early eighteenth-century, Dickens in mid-nineteenth-century and Trelawney just before the First World War, the manner in which those elements are expressed, the way in which the problems are posed and the means for their resolution, all differ from author to author and from period to period.

Again, just as the issues within nursing, including the fierce debate over registration, the monitoring of training schools for nurses, etc., were never fully resolved and continued to resurface, albeit in different guises, for the rest of the period,[59] so too is it impossible to find a nursing character or heroine who is recognisably the complete new nurse of the modern period. Perhaps the closest we may get to that prime example is the heroine of D. O. Thompson's A Dealer in Sunshine (1930), June, who chooses nursing as a career after talking to a doctor about what she should do with her life. Nursing, she was advised, had "a lot in it ... plenty of

scope and room for development, June. It's hard work and no
mere 'job' but a profession - or higher still, it's service,
June".[60]

In that novel all of the processes of recruitment, training and examination are described in detail, during which the
reader is given a clear discussion of the motivation for nursing. The middle section of the novel is taken up with the post-
graduate career choices open to June, culminating with her becoming an assistant-matron in an orphanage and eventually
matron of the orphanage. There are hints in the closing pages
of the story of a marriage between June and the hero, a young
doctor at the orphanage, but the nurse-heroine is shown as
continuing to work as a nurse. This novel, which was given as
a prize by a girls' weekly magazine, was certainly representative of a new style of treatment of the nurse in fiction, in
which the nurse/woman was depicted as a worker in her own
right and in which the heroine plays as   significant a role
in the development of the plot as the hero.[61]

That particular novel appeared at a time when young girls
were once again facing problems about their social roles, particularly regarding the relationships between work and family
life:[62] like other titles in the series, it attempted to attract women into the newer "white blouse" occupations. In its
attention to detail and despite its natural preoccupation with
romantic plot and sub-plot, A Dealer in Sunshine spelt out to
would-be nurses the conditions under which they might expect
to work and train. The desire to make explicit such statements
about nursing was set in a recurrence of the impressions that
nursing was hard, menial and unrewarding work for decent young
women, impressions which even the guides to employment of the
period failed to dispel.[63]

The need for fictional representation of nursing to closely reflect the 'realities' of nursing practice has been identified by nurses themselves, in particular by L. and E. Richter, American nurse-educators. In a recent article, (1974),
they pointed out that fiction can produce preconceptions about
practice in the minds of potential recruits which may no
longer pertain. For example, "typically, students in fiction
work long, hard hours, are often left alone at night as charge
nurses on busy floors, and live in dread of cold, harsh super-
visors whose edicts they dare not question". In order to prevent potential loss of recruits through such misrepresenta-
tions the Richters argued that nurses themselves should write
nurse-fiction, to entertain and "inspire our nurses of the future".[64]

Fiction, then, may play an important part in the production or confirmation of prejudices and beliefs and, indeed, as
Atkinson has argued,[65] fiction may actually determine behaviour
through the production of role stereotypes. In this way it is
possible to see why nurses themselves, whether like the Richters or like Nightingale and her castigation of the gamps, have

used fictional representations of themselves to develop or enhance a corporate image to which they can subscribe.

Conclusion
The history of the professions in the nineteenth- and twentieth-centuries demonstrates the ways in which practitioners altered their areas of responsibility and control in order to make their services in some way exclusive. In so doing they have transformed themselves, often literally by bringing into the occupation an entirely new group or class, or by genderising the calling as in the case of medicine, or more formally by education, training, registration and self- and State regulation.

Since such professions could not have hereditary access to knowledge or skill, entrants were literally novices, often having attributes inappropriate to the work of that group. The training system set about creating a commonly recognisable practitioner to whom the client could relate, and that training system was accompanied by rituals which the recruits and the trained professionals, as well as the clientele, could recognise as transitional stages on the road to full professional status and membership. Such progression through the ranks was marked by "rites of passage",[66] including uniforms, examinations and ceremonies, as well as earnings and the shedding of inappropriate behaviour patterns and expectations, and their replacement with socially and occupationally acceptable normative behaviour.

In nursing, as we have noted, such a process developed after the 1880's and was, while not complete, fairly well established and recognisable by 1914. The crucial relationship within nursing was that of control, whether over self or over others, and the training programme, with its discipline, set out to develop that relationship to its fullest extent. Since illness created dependency, at least physical dependency, the nurse had to learn control so that she would not exploit that dependency at the cost of the patient's comfort and well-being. At the same time, the nurse's acquisition of knowledge put her at an advantage over others, including patients, relatives and even other nurses, so that she created a psychological and social dependency in these others: her training taught her not to exploit that for her own personal ends, but only for the good of the patient, her juniors and her profession.

The two great challenges to a nurse's self-control came from her work alongside the doctor and the conflict of spheres of responsibility, and the fact that she was also a woman. The first was carefully handled by the delineation of duties in the workplace and in the training programme by the exercise of control over the syllabus by the doctors; the behaviour expected of the new nurse in the presence of the doctor, with strict application of punishment for misdemeanours, ensured its success on the wards. The second, the nurse's sexuality, was

harder to cope with within the system: it was hard to deny the
sexuality of the nurse, especially when the nurse was described as the 'handmaiden of the doctor' or as a surrogate
mother-figure. Uniforms, which obscured obvious sexual characteristics, helped, as did the chaperoning system. In the end,
both nursing and medicine recognised the need to transform
nurses from being women into members of some third gender:
doctors were expected to flirt in their early hospital life
with the nurses, just as nurses were expected to have 'crushes'
on the doctors - "every nurse is supposed to have at least one
affaire during her hospital life. It is one of the semi-
serious, wholly delightful compensations in the recognised un-
official syllabus of education; and it is perfectly understood
that in most cases it comes to nothing".[67] However, the
trained nurse, the mature woman, having been through her
training and become familiar with the intricacies of human
biology, was expected to have got over her infatuations and
be able to converse with doctors and men without the "hiatuses
essential in conversation with ordinary women": nurses were
"in the same profession as doctors" and "one could talk to
them with the same large freedom as with men".[68] Their training as new nurses made them have such a view of the world, and
of sex and gender in particular, as to make "their inherent
femininity recede into the background".[69] Nurses became, then,
not pseudo-men, semi-doctors or especially-feminine women; they
became, if they stayed in nursing, members of a "third sex"[70]
and were thus exploited twice over.[71]

NOTES

1. Abraham, Night Nurse, p. 7.
2. S. and B. Webb, State, P. 82.
3. Mrs. Bedford Fenwick, 'Nursing Echoes', British
Journal of Nursing, 29 September 1906, pp. 251-2.
4. Laurence, Nurse's Life, pp. 62-3.
5. Dr. Bedford Fenwick, Registration of Nurses, 1905,
pp. 2-3. For a recent study of skill see C. Moore, Skill and
the English Working Class, 1870 - 1914 (Croom Helm, London,
1980), pp. 15-26, pp. 41-52.
6. Carpenter, 'Asylum Nursing', p. 125.
7. For example, Loane, Englishman's Castle; M. F. Gill,
District Nursing in Brighton 1877 - 1974 (Benedict, Brighton,
1978). An introduction to some of these other groups is given
in B. Ehrenreich and D. English, Witches, Midwives and Nurses:
A History of Women Healers (Writers and Readers Publishing
Cooperative, London, 1976) and M. C. Vesluysen, 'Old Wives'
Tales? Women Healers in English History' in Davies (editor),
Rewriting, pp. 175-199.
8. For an introduction to the use of such material see,
Basch, Relative Creatures, pp. xviii - xx; Spearman, 'Fiction';
Spearman, Novel and Society; Cazamain, Social Novel, pp. 7-11;

J. Rockwell, Fact in Fiction: The Use of Literature in the systematic study of society (Routledge and Kegan Paul, London, 1974), Chapters 1 - 3; P. Thomson, The Victorian Heroine: A Changing Ideal 1837 - 1873 (O. U. P., London, 1956). For a cautionary note about fiction and women's roles see, Branca, Silent Sisterhood, pp. 11-12. However, "Thackeray confessed that men and women in novels had to be represented according to current convention". C. Pearl, The Girl with the Swansdown Seat (Muller, London, 1955), p. 6.

    9. Basch, Relative Creatures, pp. 145-6, pp. 182-3.

    10. R. Hoggart, The Uses of Literacy (Chatto and Windus, London, 1957) (1969 edition), p. 206; Basch, Relative Creatures, pp. xix - xx, pp. 272-74.

    11. Rockwell, Fact in Fiction, p. 4.

    12. R. Williams, Culture and Society 1780 - 1950, (Chatto and Windus, London, 1958) (1961 edition), p. 99.

    13. Abel-Smith, Nursing Profession, p. 1. See also, Vaizey, Institutional Life, Dedication, np.

    14. Nightingale, Notes on Nursing, (1859).

    15. Ibid., Preface, np.

    16. Nightingale, 'Training of Nurses', p. 237.

    17. D. Defoe, A Journal of the Plague Year (1722) (Dent, London, 1966, edition), pp. 93-5.

    18. Ibid., p. 96.

    19. Ibid., p. ix.

    20. Ibid., p. 101. The class of patient recurs in the novels surveyed here: see, for example, Mrs. Humphrey Ward, Marcella (Smith, Elder, London, 1894). Providing nurses for the poorer classes was, of course, a major preoccupation for nurse-reformers including Nightingale, Agnes Jones and Elizabeth Fry.

    21. F. J. Gant, 'Satan in Petticoats: The Husband Huntress and Trapper Nurse', Medical Press and Circular, 11 November 1899, pp. 395-6. The vampyre motif is fully discussed in C. J. Frayling (editor), The Vampyre: Lord Ruthven to Count Dracula (Gollancz, London, 1978).

    22. Trelawney, Cottage Hospital, p. vii.

    23. Abraham, Night Nurse, p. 131.

    24. Basch, Relative Creatures, pp. 144-6. A similar criticism may be levelled at Dickens's caricatures of the new sciences; for example, mathematics and Mr. Gradgrind, in Hard Times (1854). See, Williams, Culture and Society, pp. 104-108. As Pearl has noted, "Dickens, despite his satire, despite his eldest son at Eton, despite his mistress, is the voice of middle-class England". Pearl, Swansdown Seat, p. 14, p. 30, p. 66. See also the idea of necrophilia and Sarah Gamp in Basch, Relative Creatures, p. 146.

    25. For example, the opinion of a servant girl - "She's an artful one, she is, with all her demure looks and mincing ways. I'm not blind. Only comes here because she can wear them play-acting clothes and show off. I haven't the patience with

her. Lady-nurse, indeed. No more a lady than I am". Also, a footman and coachman - "Regular nurse, ain't she?, said the coachman, Horspittle? Yes, I suppose so. Dressed up like a nun out for a holiday. Why couldn't they have had a nurse out of the village, or your wife?" G. M. Fenn, <u>Nurse Elisia</u> (Hurst and Blackett, London, 1893), pp. 54-5, p. 221.

    26. A. Trollope, <u>Orley Farm</u> (Collins, London, 1862), cited in Thomson, <u>Victorian Heroine</u>, p. 73. For a comparison with Nightingale's own life see, Woodham-Smith, <u>Florence Nightingale</u>, pp. 48-99, pp. 66-7.

    27. R. N. Carey, <u>Merle's Crusade</u> (Religious Tract Society, London, 1889), pp. 30-1.

    28. Ibid., p. 31.

    29. Basch, <u>Relative Creatures</u>, p. 190.

    30. Ibid., p.183.

    31. Nightingale, <u>Notes on Nursing</u>, Preface, np.

    32. Ward, <u>Marcella</u>, p. 259.

    33. Cunningham, 'New Woman'; L. Fernando, <u>New Women in the Late Victorian Novel</u> (Pennsylvania State University Press, London, 1977); L. Dowling, 'The Decadent and the New Woman in the 1890's', <u>Nineteenth-Century Fiction</u>, 33, 4 March 1979, pp. 434-53.

    34. Abraham, <u>Night Nurse</u>, p. 6.

    35. Needham and Utter, <u>Pamela's Daughters</u>, p. 339.

    36. Abraham, <u>Night Nurse</u>, pp. 75-6.

    37. Ibid., p. 95.

    38. C. Dickens, <u>Martin Chuzzlewit</u> (1843/4) (Hazell, Watson and Viney, London, nd.), pp. 342-3.

    39. Ward, <u>Marcella</u>, p. 302.

    40. Basch, <u>Relative Creatures</u>, p. 145.

    41. Pearl, <u>Swansdown Seat</u>, p. 30.

    42. For contemporary criticisms of asylums see, R. Z. Dale, <u>In a County Asylum</u> (Werner Laurie, London, nd.); J. W. Cobbett, 'How Insanity is Propagated', <u>Westminster Review</u>, 1894, 142 (2), pp. 153-63; J.W. Cobbett, 'Ought Private Lunatic Asylums to be Abolished?', <u>Westminster Review</u>, 1894, 142, (4), pp. 369-80. See also A. T. Scull, <u>Museums of Madness: The Social Organisation of Insanity in Nineteenth-Century England</u> (Lane, London, 1979).

    43. C. Reade, <u>Hard Cash</u> (Chatto and Windus, London, 1863) (1899 edition), p. 446.

    44. Ibid., p. 447.

    45. Ibid., p. 360.

    46. Brightfield, 'Medical Profession', pp. 238-56.

    47. C. Bronte, <u>Shirley</u> (1849) (Penguin, London, 1979 edition), p. 526.

    48. S. and B. Webb, <u>State</u>, p. 82.

    49. Ward, <u>Marcella</u>, p. 302.

    50. Ibid., pp. 307-8.

    51. Ibid., pp. 304-5.

    52. Ibid., p. 306.

53. Munro, Science, p. 4.

54. Trelawney, Cottage Hospital, p. 65. Compare this be-haviour with that of Marcella and Sarah Gamp.

55. Ibid., pp. 75-6.

56. Maule, 'Training Schools', p. 57.

57. Nightingale, 'Training of Nurses', p. 244. Compare these with prison officer virtues; see Chapter 3, footnote, 66.

58. Ignatieff, Just Measure of Pain, pp. 103-4.

59. For an overview see, Baly, Nursing and Social Change.

60. D. O. Thompson, A Dealer in Sunshine (Every Girls Paper Office, London, 1930), p. 20. See also, Carey, Merle's Crusade, pp. 30-1.

61. See also the Sue Barton and the Cherry Ames series from America. H. Boylson, Sue Barton (1936-52); H. Wells and T. Tatham, Cherry Ames (1944 -). For a comment on this depar-ture see, L. Richter and E. Richter, 'Nurses in Fiction', American Journal of Nursing, July 1974, p. 1281; Neff, Vic-torian Working Women, pp. 253-4.

62. Taylor, 'Daughters and Mothers', pp. 122-3.

63. Strachey, Careers, pp. 56-60.

64. Richter and Richter, 'Nurses in Fiction', p. 1281.

65. P. Atkinson, 'Kind Hearts and Curettes', New Society, 27 July 1972, p. 178.

66. A. Van Gennep, The Rites of Passage (Routledge and Kegan Paul, London, 1960) (1965 edition), p. 103.

67. Abraham, Night Nurse, p. 198.

68. Ibid., p. 102.

69. Ibid., p. 102.

70. Ibid., p. 102.

71. That is, once as nurses and once as women. See Gamarnikow, 'Sexual Division of Labour', pp. 114-117.

SELECT BIBLIOGRAPHY

A complete bibliography is given in C. Maggs, 'Aspects of the
Recruitment, Training and Post-Certification Experiences of
General Hospital Nurses in England 1881 - 1914, Ph.D., Univer-
sity of Bath, 1980.

Government Publications

Select Committee on the Metropolitan Hospitals, PP 1890/1,
   xiii
Select Committee on Registration of Nurses, PP 1904, vi
Select Committee on Registration of Nurses, PP 1905, vii
Royal Commission on the Poor Laws, PP 1909, xxxvii
Census of Population, 1921

Journals

American Journal of Nursing
British Journal of Nursing
The Hospital
The Lancet
Medical Press and Circular
Nursing Mirror
Nursing Record
Nursing Times
Nursing World and Hospital Review
Poor Law Officers Journal
Trained Nurse and Hospital Review
Westminster Review

Books, Articles and Theses

B. Abel-Smith, A History of the Nursing Profession (Heinemann,
   London, 1960)
J. J. Abraham, The Night Nurse (Chapman and Hall, London,
   1913)
G. Anderson, Victorian Clerks (Manchester University Press,
   Manchester, 1976)
   —— 'The Social Economy of Late Victorian Clerks' in G.
   Crossick (editor), The Lower Middle Class in Britain 1870 -
   1914 (Croom Helm, London, 1977)

P. Atkinson, Kind Hearts and Curettes, New Society, 27 July 1972
E. Bagnold, A Diary Without Dates (Heinemann, London, 1918)
H. Balme, A Criticism of Nurse Education (Oxford University Press, Oxford, 1937)
M. Baly, Nursing and Social Change (Heinemann, London, 1973)
J. A. Banks, Prosperity and Parenthood (Schoken, London, 1954)
E. Barritt, 'Florence Nightingale's Values and Modern Nursing Education', Nursing Forum, 12, 1, 1973
E. C. Barton, The History and Progress of Poor Law Nursing (Law and Local Government Publications, London, 1926)
F. Basch, Relative Creatures (Allen, Lane, London, 1974)
P. Branca, 'Image and Reality: The Myth of the Idle Victorian Woman' in M. Hartman and L. W. Banner (editors), Clio's Consciousness Raised (Harper, New York, 1974)
—— Silent Sisterhood (Croom Helm, London, 1975)
—— Women in Europe since 1750 (Croom Helm, London, 1978)
M. J. Brightfield, 'The Medical Profession in Early Victorian England as depicted in the novels of the period 1840 - 1870', Bulletin of the History of Medicine, XXXV, 1961
V. Brittain, Testament of Youth (Gollancz, London, 1933)
W. Brockbank, The History of Nursing at the Manchester Royal Infirmary (Manchester University Press, Manchester, 1970)
C. Bronte, Shirley, (1849) (Penguin, London, 1979)
F. F. Brooks, Nursing in Many Fields (Johnson, London, 1977)
L. Broom and J. H . Smith, 'Bridging Occupations', British Journal of Sociology, XLV, (4), December 1963
H. C. Burdett, Hospitals and the State (Churchill, London, 1881)
—— Hints in Sickness: Where to Go and What to Do (Kegan Paul, Trench, London, 1883)
—— Burdett's Official Directory of Nurses (Scientific Press, London, 1898)
—— The Nursing Profession: How and Where to Train (Scientific Press, London, 1899)
—— How to Succeed as a Trained Nurse (Scientific Press, London, 1913)
R. N. Carey, Merle's Crusade (Religious Tract Society, London, 1889)
M. Carpenter, 'The New Managerialism and Professionalism in Nursing' in M. Stacey et al (editors), Health Care and the Division of Labour (Croom Helm, London, 1977)
—— 'Asylum Nursing before 1914: A Chapter in the History of Labour' in C.Davies (editor), Rewriting Nursing History (Croom Helm, London, 1980)
S.B. Carter, A New Deal for Nurses (Gollancz, London, 1939)
L. Cazamain, The Social Novel in England 1830 - 1850 (Routledge and Kegan Paul, London, 1973)
C. Collet, 'The Collection and Utilisation of Official Statistics bearing on the extent and effects of the Industrial Employment of Women', Journal of the Royal Statistical

Society, LXI, Part II, June 1898

A. R. Cunningham, 'The 'New Women' Fiction of the 1890's', Victorian Studies, 17 December 1973

E. Davidson, 'A Career in Nursing a Century Ago', Nursing Mirror, 13 April 1978

C. Davies, 'Experiences of Dependency and Control in Work', Journal of Advanced Nursing, 1, 1976

——— 'Continuities in the Development of Hospital Nursing in Britain', Journal of Advanced Nursing, 2, 1977

——— 'Professionalizing Strategies as Time- and Culture-Bound: The Case of American nursing circa 1893' unpublished paper, B.S.A. Medical Sociology Conference, York, 1978

——— 'Where Next for Nursing History?', Nursing Times, 22 May 1980

——— 'The Contemporary Challenge in Nursing History' in C. Davies (editor), Rewriting Nursing History (Croom Helm, London, 1980)

——— Rewriting Nursing History (Croom Helm, London, 1980)

——— 'A Constant Casualty: Nurse Education in Britain and the U.S.A. to 1939' in C. Davies, Rewriting Nursing History (Croom Helm, London, 1980)

——— 'The Regulation of Nursing Work: An Historical Comparison of Britain and the U.S.A.', Research in the Sociology of Health Care, Vol. 2, 1982

A. Davin, 'Telegraphists and Clerks', Bulletin of the Society for the Study of Labour History, 26, Spring 1973

M. Dean and G. Bolton, 'The Administration of Poverty and the Development of Nursing Practice in Britain in Nineteenth-Century England' in C. Davies (editor), Rewriting Nursing History, (Croom Helm, London, 1980)

D. Defoe, A Journal of the Plague Year (1722) (Dent, London, 1977)

C. Dickens, Martin Chuzzlewit (1843/4) (Hazell, Watson and Viney, London, nd.)

M. Dickens, One Pair of Feet (Penguin, London, 1980)

Lady Dilke et al (editors), Women's Work (Methuen, London, 1894)

J. Donnison, Midwives and Medical Men (Heinemann, London, 1977)

L. Dowling, 'The Decadent and the New Woman in the 1890's', Nineteenth-Century Fiction, 33, 4 March 1979

D. Dunkerly, Occupations and Society (Routledge and Kegan Paul, London, 1975)

M. Ebery and B. Preston, Domestic Service in Late Victorian and Edwardian England 1871 - 1914 (University of Reading, Reading, 1976)

G. M. Fenn, Nurse Elisia (Hurst and Blackett, London, 1893)

J. Floud and W. Scott, 'Recruitment in Teaching in England and Wales' in A. H. Halsey, J. Floud and C. A. Anderson (editors), Education, Economics and Society (Free Press, New York, 1961)

E. Gamarnikow, 'The Sexual Division of Labour: The Case of

Nursing' in A.Kuhn and A. M. Wolpe (editors), <u>Feminism and Materialism</u> (Routledge, London, 1978)

F. Gilpin, <u>Scenes from Hospital Life</u> (Drane, London, nd.)

A. W. Goodrich, <u>The Social and Ethical Significance of Nursing</u> (MacMillan, New York, 1932)

Guy's Hospital, <u>Nursing Guide</u> (Ash, London, 1904)

A. Hake, <u>Suffering London</u> (Scientific Press, London, 1892)

G. M. Hardy, <u>Yes, Matron</u> (Beck, London, 1951)

B. Harrison, 'Oral History and Recent Political History', <u>Oral History</u>, 3, 1973

W. Hector, <u>Mrs. Bedford Fenwick</u> (R. C. N., London, 1973)

S. Hogg, 'The Employment of Women in Great Britain 1891 - 1921', D.Phil., University of Oxford, 1964

L. Holcombe, <u>Victorian Ladies at Work</u> (David and Charles, Newton Abbot, 1973)

P. Horn, <u>The Rise and Fall of the Victorian Servant</u> (Gill and MacMillan, Dublin, 1975)

B. Howe, <u>A Galaxy of Governesses</u> (Yerschoyle, London, 1959)

M. Ignatieff, <u>A Just Measure of Pain</u> (MacMillan, London, 1978)

F. Jarman, 'The Development of Conceptions of Nursing Professionalism among General Hospital Nurses 1860 - 1895', M.A., University of Warwick, 1980

Lady S. M. Jeune (editor), <u>Ladies at Work</u> (Arnold, London, 1893)

P. Kalisch and B. Kalisch, <u>The Advance of American Nursing</u> (Little, Boston, U.S.A., 1978)

E. C. Laurence, <u>A Nurse's Life in War and Peace</u> (Smith, Elder, London, 1912)

P. G.Lewis, <u>Theory and Practice of Nursing</u> (Scientific Press, London, 1893)

E. Luckes, <u>Hospital Sisters and Their Duties</u> (Churchill, London, 1886)

────── What Will Trained Nurses gain by joining the British Nurse's Association? (Churchill, London, 1889)

────── <u>General Nursing</u> (Kegan Paul, Trench and Trubner, London, 1898)

C. Maggs, 'Control Mechanisms and the 'new nurses' 1881 - 1914', <u>Nursing Times</u>, 2 September 1981

G. M. Mercer, <u>The Employment of Nurses: Nursing Labour Turnover in the National Health Service</u> (Croom Helm, London, 1979)

C. Moore, <u>Skill and the English Working Class, 1870 - 1914</u> (Croom Helm, London, 1980)

H. Morten, <u>How to Become a Nurse</u> (Scientific Press, London, 1895)

P. E. Moulder, 'The General Servant Problem', <u>Westminster Review</u>, CLX, August 1903

A. Munro, <u>The Science and Art of Nursing the Sick</u> (Maclehouse, Glasgow, 1873)

T. McBride, <u>The Domestic Revolution</u> (Croom Helm, London, 1976)

R. Nash (editor), <u>Florence Nightingale to Her Nurses</u>

(MacMillan, London, 1914)

W. Neff, <u>Victorian Working Women</u> (Allen and Unwin, London, 1966)

R. Nettleton, 'A Nurse's Life in the 1900's, <u>Nursing Times</u>, 21 December 1972

Florence Nightingale, <u>Notes on Nursing</u> (1860) (Morris,London, 1946 reprint)

———— 'The Training of Nurses and Nursing the Sick Poor' in R. Quain (editor), <u>Dictionary of Medicine</u> (Longmans Green, London, 1882)

A. Oram, 'The Employment of Women Teachers 1910 - 1938', unpublished paper, University of Bristol, 1978

N. Parry and J. Parry, <u>The Rise of the Medical Profession</u> (Croom Helm, London, 1976)

G. Partington, <u>Women Teachers in the 20th Century in England and Wales</u> (N.F.E.R. Publishing, London, 1976)

C. Pearl, <u>The Girl with the Swansdown Seat</u> (Muller, London, 1955)

M. J. Peterson, <u>The Medical Profession in Mid-Victorian London</u> (University of California Press, London, 1978)

Mrs. Phillips (editor), <u>A Dictionary of Employment Open to Women</u> (Women's Institute, London, 1898)

M. Phillips and W. S. Tomkinson, <u>English Women in Life and Letters: Women in the Professions</u> (O.U.P., Oxford, 1927)

R. Pinker, <u>English Hospital Statistics 1861 - 1938</u> (Heinemann, London, 1966)

S. Pollard, <u>The Genesis of Modern Management</u> (Arnold, London, 1965)

G. W. Potter, <u>Ministering Women: TheStory of the Royal National Pension Fund for Nurses</u> (The Hospital, London, 1891)

F. N. L. Poynter (editor), <u>The Evolution of Hospitals in Britain</u> (Pitman, London, 1964)

C. Reade, <u>Hard Cash</u> (Chatto and Windus, London, 1863)

L. Richter and E. Richter, 'Nurses in Fiction', <u>American Journal of Nursing</u>, July 1974

J. Rockwell, <u>Fact in Fiction</u> (Routledge and Kegan Paul, London, 1974)

G. Saleeby, <u>Woman and Womanhood</u> (Heinemann, London, 1909)

R. Samuel, 'Local History and Oral History', <u>History Workshop</u>, 1, 1976

J. Saville, <u>Rural Depopulation in England and Wales</u> (Routledge and Kegan Paul, London, 1957)

M. Schofield, 'On a Summer's Day in 1879', <u>Nursing Mirror</u>, 4 June 1971

A. T.Scull, <u>Museums of Madness</u> (Allen Lane, London, 1979)

L. Seymer (editor), <u>Selected·Writings of Florence Nightingale</u> (MacMillan, New York, 1954)

———— <u>Florence Nightingale's Nurses: The Nightingale Training School 1860 - 1960</u> (Pitman, London, 1960)

H. M. Simpson, 'The Influence of Professional Nursing on the Development of the Modern Hospital' in Poynter (editor), <u>The</u>

Evolution of Hospitals

F. B. Smith, The People's Health 1830 - 1910 (Croom Helm, London, 1979)

——— Florence Nightingale: Reputation and Power (Croom Helm, London, 1982)

D. Spearman, The Novel and Society (Routledge and Kegan Paul, London, 1966)

——— 'The Social Influence of Fiction', New Society, 6 July 1972

M. Stollard, 'Nursing on £12 a year', Yorkshire Post, 7 May 1962

R. Strachey, Careers and Opportunities for Women (Faber and Faber, London, 1935)

P. Stubbs, Women and Fiction: Feminism and the Novel 1880 - 1920 (Harvester, Sussex, 1979)

P. Taylor, 'Daughters and Mothers - maids and mistresses: Domestic Service between the Wars' in J. Clarke et al (editors), Working-Class Culture: Studies in History and Theory (Hutchinson, London, 1979)

A. Terton, Lights and Shadows in a Hospital (Methuen, London, 1902)

D. O. Thompson, A Dealer in Sunshine (Every Girl's Paper Office, London, 1930)

E. P. Thompson, 'Time, Work-Discipline and Industrial Capitalism', Past and Present, 38, 1967

P. Thompson, The Voice of the Past: Oral History (O.U.P., London, 1978)

P. Thomson, The Victorian Heroine: A Changing Ideal 1837 - 1873 (O. U. P., London, 1956)

S. A. Tooley, The History of Nursing in the British Empire (Bonsfield, London, 1906)

G. Trelawney, In A Cottage Hospital (Werner Laurie, London, 1901)

A. Tropp, The School Teachers (Heinemann, London, 1957)

(Various authors), The Science and Art of Nursing (Cassells, London, 1908)

M. Vivian, Lectures to Nurses in Training (Scientific Press, London, 1920)

M. Voysey, Nursing: Hints to Probationers on Practical Work (Scientific Press, London, 1901)

Mrs. Humphrey Ward, Marcella (Smith, Elder, London, 1894)

B. Webb, 'English Teachers and Their Professional Organisation', New Statesman, Special Supplements, 1915

S. and B. Webb, The State and the Doctor (Longmans Green, London, 1910)

R. White, 'Some Political Influences surrounding the Nurses Registration Act 1919 in the United Kingdom', Journal of Advanced Nursing, 1, 1976

——— 'The Development of the Poor Law Nursing Service 1848 - 1948: A Discussion of the Historical Method and a Summary of some of the Findings', International Journal of Nursing

Studies, 14, (1), 1977
——— Social Change and the Development of the Nursing Profession (Kimpton, London, 1978)
W. Whittall, Pensions for Hospital Officers and Staffs (Layton, London, 1919)
F. Widdowson, Going Up Into The Next Class: Women and Elementary Teacher Training 1840 - 1916 (W.R.R.C., London, 1980)
K. Williams, 'From Sarah Gamp to Florence Nightingale: A Critical Study of Hospital Nursing Systems from 1840 to 1897' in Davies (editor), Rewriting Nursing History
E. Wilson, Gone with the Raj (Reeve, Norfolk, 1974)
C. Woodham-Smith, Florence Nightingale (Constable, London, 1950)
J. Woodward, To Do The Sick No Harm: A Study of the British Voluntary Hospital System to 1875 (Routledge and Kegan Paul, London, 1974)
V. Young, Outlines of Nursing (Scientific Press, London, 1914)

Oral Evidence (unpublished)

Interviews carried out 1977 - 79 with

Mrs. Davies
Mrs. Elton
Mrs. Evenden
Mrs. Foster
Mrs. Gibbons
Mrs. Hawke

Mrs. Hitchin
Mrs. Kemp
Mrs. Kenwell
Mrs. Maden
Mrs. McLellan
Mrs. O'Keefe

Mrs. Pearce
Mrs. Richards
Miss Ryder
Miss Spyer
Mrs. W.

eight-hour day 95
elementary schoolteachers
42, 51-7, 69, 75, 116;
and nursing 42, 54, 56,
57, 69, 75
entrance test 20-1, 82
eugenics 14, 157-8
'everywoman is a nurse'
11, 88, 102, 149, 151,
154, 155
exploitation, dependency
and 12-13, 137-8, 148-
51, 153, 158, 159-60,
163-4, 165, 167

family imagery in nursing
11-12, 13-14, 17, 97,
115, 120, 134-5, 138,
148-9, 155, 168
Fenn, G. M. 152
Fenwick, Dr. Bedford: evolution of nursing 5, 63;
on registration 12-13,
117
Fenwick, Mrs. Bedford: on
lady-pupils 146; on
registration 12-13, 117
on type of recruit 38
fiction as source 28, 30-1,
148, 149, 166-7
fictional nurses 11, 13,
15, 89, 91, 148, 149-50,
166-7; as vampires 151-
3, 168; Betsy Prig 17,
153, 158; June 165-6;
Marcella 161-2; May Pat-
terson 152; Merle 155;
motives of 155-6, 157;
Nurse Elisia 149, 154;
Nurse Hannah 160; Ruth
156; Sarah (Sairey) Gamp
17, 30, 153, 158; work of
150, 153, 158-9, 163-4,
166; Zillah Horsfall 154,
160-1

Gaskell, Elizabeth 148, 156
general hospital nurses: as
third sex 145, 167-8;
careers of 98, 118, 120-5,
128-30, 131-5; contribution

to health 1, 5, 9-10, 137-
8; costs of 120, 125-8,
130; definitions of 1-2,
14-15; need for 6, 88,
137-8, 145; numbers of 7-
9, 119-20; pensions and
130-1; registers of 116-8;
supremacy of 1, 26-8, 115-
6, 123, 125, 132, 136, 137-
9; work of 9, 123, 145,
147
Ginsberg, E. 75

Haycraft, Mrs. 152
historiography of nursing
2-3, 6, 147-8
hospitals: beds in 6-7, 73;
Brownlow Hill 78; Chelsea
Poor Law Infirmary 20;
cottage 7, 135, 136; general hospitals 1-2, 6, 10,
12, 16, 19, 28, 63, 88, 103,
145; growth of 1, 5, 6-7,
14; Guy's 78, 91, 93, 128;
King's College 10, 125;
Leeds General Infirmary
78, 95; Leeds Poor Law Infirmary 29; length of stay
in 9-10; Liverpool Royal
Infirmary 78; Manchester
Royal Infirmary 20, 23,
29, 82, 95, 98, 131; Mid-
dlesex 119, 146; Poor Law
1, 6, 27, 71, 78, 100, 118-
9, 133-4, 137; Poplar and
Stepney Sick Asylum 29,
77-8, 84; Portsmouth Poor
Law Infirmary 29, 71; re-
cords of 28-9, 31, 118,
134; Royal Hants Infirmary
29; Royal South Hants In-
firmary 29, 78; Salisbury
General Infirmary 29;
Southampton Poor Law In-
firmary 29, 118; St. Bar-
tholomew's 63, 123, 131;
St. Thomas's 10, 97, 101,
103, 165; The London 29,
73, 78, 92, 97, 117, 118;
type of patient in 1-2, 12,
28, 108, 130, 137-8; volun-

ward work   24-5, 91, 92-3
White, R.   10
women's work: changes in   11,
   12, 31, 38, 39, 42, 44-5,
   46, 51-2, 68, 74, 135, 154-
   5, 165; 'white-blouse'   14,
   38, 42, 49-57, 68-9, 135